Subject labels and numbered tabs are located at the end of the book. Either place the subject labels to the right or write in your own topics. Then apply the numbered tabs to the corresponding pages.

1.

☞ P9-DHJ-251

2. _____

→

3. _____

→

4. _____

→

5. _____

→

6. _____

→

7. _____

→

8. _____

→

9. _____

→

10. _____

→

11. _____

→

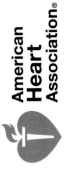

American
Heart
Association®

2010 Handbook of
Emergency
Cardiovascular Care

for Healthcare Providers

Editors

Mary Fran Hazinski, RN, MSN
Ricardo Samson, MD
Steve Schexnayder, MD

Senior Managing Editor

Jennifer Ashcraft, RN, BSN

Reviewed by the members of

Committee on Emergency Cardiovascular Care
Subcommittee on Basic Life Support
Subcommittee on Pediatric Resuscitation
Subcommittee on Advanced Cardiovascular Life Support

With materials adapted from

2010 AHA Guidelines for CPR and ECC
Basic Life Support for Healthcare Providers
Pediatric Advanced Life Support
Neonatal Resuscitation Textbook
Advanced Cardiovascular Life Support
ILCOR Advisory Statements
ACC/AHA Guidelines for Management
of ACS (2005-2010)

Additional contributions from

Clifton W. Callaway, MD, PhD
Elizabeth Sinz, MD
Sallie Young, PharmD, BCPS,
Pharmacotherapy Editor

Preface

This 2010 edition of the *Handbook of Emergency Cardiovascular Care for Healthcare Providers* provides our readers with the latest recommendations from the 2010 American Heart Association Guidelines for Cardiopulmonary Resuscitation and Emergency Cardiovascular Care. The Guidelines represent the best current understanding of science and translation of the science into direct patient care. The material in this handbook was selected for its relevance to patient care and its application to a quick-reference format. While these recommendations are founded in an extensive international science review, not all recommendations will apply to all rescuers and all victims in all situations. The leader of the resuscitation may need to adapt the application of these recommendations to unique circumstances.

The 2010 AHA Guidelines for CPR and ECC mark the 50th year since the publication of the landmark article by Kouwenhoven, Jude, and Knickerbocker reporting successful closed chest compressions. The resuscitation community also celebrates recent reports of increased survival from cardiac arrest with focus on provision of high-quality CPR and postarrest support. With such efforts, as well as a continued commitment to the advancement of resuscitation science, thousands of lives can be saved every year.

Mary Fran Hazinski
Steve Schexnayder
Ricardo Samson

Note on Medication Doses

Emergency cardiovascular care is a dynamic science. Advances in treatment and drug therapies occur rapidly. Readers are advised to check for changes in recommended dose, indications, and contraindications in the following sources: future editions of this handbook and AHA training materials, as well as the package insert product information sheet for each drug.

Clinical condition and pharmacokinetics may require drug dose or interval dosing adjustments. Specific parameters may require monitoring, for example, of creatinine clearance or QT interval. Some medications listed in this handbook may not be available in all countries, and may not be specifically approved by regulatory agencies in some countries for a particular indication.

Special Acknowledgment

We offer special thanks to Brenda Schoolfield for her extraordinary efforts and contributions to the timely revision of this 2010 Handbook.

Copyright Notice

Contents

iii

Basic Life Support for Healthcare Providers

Recognition and Activation/CPR and Rescue Breathing/Defibrillation

The following sequence is intended for a single healthcare provider rescuer. If additional rescuers are available, the first rescuer feels for a pulse for no more than 10 seconds and starts chest compressions if the pulse is not definitely palpated. A second rescuer activates the emergency response number and obtains an automated external defibrillator (AED), and a third rescuer opens the airway and provides ventilation.

Recognition and Activation

Victim is unresponsive; the adult is not breathing or not breathing normally (ie, agonal gasps), and the infant or child is not breathing or only gasping.

Activate emergency response system or appropriate resuscitation team.

Pulse Check

Check for pulse for no more than 10 seconds (carotid in adult; carotid or femoral in child; brachial in infant).

- **If pulse absent:** Provide CPR (start with chest compressions and perform cycles of 30 compressions and 2 breaths) until AED or advanced life support (ALS) providers arrive. For 2 rescuers, the compression-ventilation ratio for infants and children (to the age of puberty) is 15:2.

- **If pulse present** but breathing is absent, open the airway and provide rescue breathing (1 breath every 5 to 6 seconds for adult, 1 breath every 3 to 5 seconds for infant or child). Recheck pulse about every 2 minutes.

- **In infant or child with adequate oxygenation and ventilation if pulse present but <60/min with poor perfusion:** Begin chest compressions with ventilations.

CPR (C-A-B)

C. Compressions
Begin CPR with 30 chest compressions. (If 2 rescuers for infant or child, provide 15 compressions.)

A. Open airway
After chest compressions, open airway with head tilt–chin lift or jaw thrust.

B. Breathing
- *If victim is breathing* or resumes effective breathing, place in the recovery position.
- *If victim is not breathing,* give 2 breaths that make chest rise. Release completely; allow for exhalation between breaths. After 2 breaths, immediately resume chest compressions.

Continue Basic Life Support Until More Skilled Providers Arrive
Integrate newborn resuscitation, pediatric advanced life support, or advanced cardiovascular life support at earliest opportunity.

Defibrillation
Defibrillation with AEDs is an integral part of basic life support.

Summary of BLS Maneuvers for Adults, Children, and Infants

Component	Recommendations		
	Adults	**Children**	**Infants**
Recognition	Unresponsive (for all ages)		
	No breathing or no normal breathing (ie, only gasping)	No breathing or only gasping	
	No pulse palpated within 10 seconds		
CPR Sequence	C-A-B		
Compression Rate	At least 100/min		
Compression Depth	At least 2 inches (5 cm)	At least ⅓ AP diameter About 2 inches (5 cm)	At least ⅓ AP diameter About 1½ inches (4 cm)
Chest Wall Recoil	Allow complete recoil between compressions Rotate compressors every 2 minutes		

Compression Interruptions	Minimize interruptions in chest compressions Attempt to limit interruptions to <10 seconds	
Airway	Head tilt–chin lift (suspected trauma: jaw thrust)	
Compression-to-Ventilation Ratio (until advanced airway placed)	30:2 1 or 2 rescuers	30:2 Single rescuer 15:2 2 rescuers
Ventilations With Advanced Airway	1 breath every 6-8 seconds (8-10 breaths/min) Asynchronous with chest compressions About 1 second per breath Visible chest rise	
Defibrillation	Attach and use AED as soon as available. Minimize interruptions in chest compressions before and after shock; resume CPR beginning with compressions immediately after each shock.	

Abbreviations: AED, automated external defibrillator; AP, anterior-posterior; CPR, cardiopulmonary resuscitation.

2

BLS Adult HCP Algorithm*

Recommendations for CPR Before Insertion of an Advanced Airway

During 2-rescuer CPR when there is no advanced airway in place, rescuers perform cycles of 30 compressions and 2 breaths. The compressor pauses after every 30 compressions to allow delivery of 2 rescue breaths. Rescuers should change compressor role every 5 cycles or 2 minutes. Rescuers should try to change compressor role in <5 seconds.

Unresponsive
No breathing or no normal breathing (ie, only gasping)

↓

Activate emergency response system
Get AED/defibrillator
or send second rescuer (if available) to do this

↓

Check pulse: DEFINITE pulse within 10 seconds?

Definite Pulse →
- **Give 1 breath every 5 to 6 seconds**
- **Recheck pulse every 2 minutes**

No Pulse ↓

Begin cycles of 30 **COMPRESSIONS** and 2 **BREATHS**

High-Quality CPR
- Rate at least 100/min
- Compression depth at least 2 inches (5 cm)
- Allow complete chest recoil after each compression
- Minimize interruptions in chest compressions
- Avoid excessive ventilation

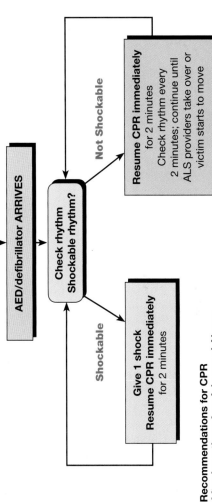

AED/defibrillator ARRIVES

Check rhythm
Shockable rhythm?

Shockable

Give 1 shock
Resume CPR immediately
for 2 minutes

Not Shockable

Resume CPR immediately
for 2 minutes
Check rhythm every
2 minutes; continue until
ALS providers take over or
victim starts to move

Recommendations for CPR
After Insertion of an Advanced Airway

Once an advanced airway is in place, 2 rescuers no longer deliver "cycles" of CPR (compressions interrupted by pauses for ventilation). Instead, the compressing rescuer should give continuous chest compressions at a rate of at least 100/min without pauses for ventilation. The rescuer delivering ventilation provides 1 breath every 6 to 8 seconds. Two or more rescuers should change compressor role approximately every 2 minutes to prevent compressor fatigue and deterioration in quality and rate of chest compressions given. Rescuers should try to change compressor role in <5 seconds.

³

*The boxes bordered with dashed lines are performed by healthcare providers and not by lay rescuers.

Simplified BLS Adult Algorithm

Unresponsive
No breathing or
no normal breathing
(only gasping)

Activate
emergency
response

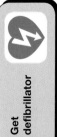

Get
defibrillator

Start CPR

Check rhythm/
shock if
indicated

Repeat every 2 minutes

Push Hard • Push Fast

4

Basic Life Support for Healthcare Providers

Relief of Foreign-Body Airway Obstruction

Adult (Adolescent [puberty] and older)	Child (1 year to adolescent [puberty])	Infant (Less than 1 year of age)
1. Ask "Are you choking?"	1. Ask "Are you choking?"	1. Confirm severe airway obstruction. Check for sudden onset of severe breathing difficulty, ineffective or silent cough, weak or silent cry.
2. Give abdominal thrusts/Heimlich maneuver or chest thrusts for pregnant or obese victims.	2. Give abdominal thrusts/Heimlich maneuver.	2. Give up to 5 back slaps *and* up to 5 chest thrusts.
3. Repeat abdominal thrusts (or chest thrusts if victim is pregnant or obese) until effective or victim becomes unresponsive.	3. Repeat abdominal thrusts until effective or victim becomes unresponsive.	3. Repeat step 2 until effective or victim becomes unresponsive.

Victim becomes unresponsive

4. Send someone to activate emergency response system.
5. Lower victim to floor. If victim is unresponsive with no breathing or no normal breathing (ie, agonal gasps), begin CPR (no pulse check).
6. Before you deliver breaths, look into mouth. If you see a foreign body that can be easily removed, remove it.
7. Continue CPR for 5 cycles or about 2 minutes. If you are alone, activate EMS system. Return and continue CPR until more skilled rescuers arrive.

Refer to BLS for Healthcare Providers course materials for more information about relief of foreign-body airway obstruction.

Building Blocks of CPR

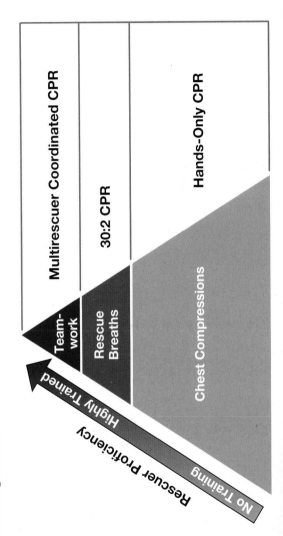

Cardiac Arrest Algorithm

Shout for Help/Activate Emergency Response

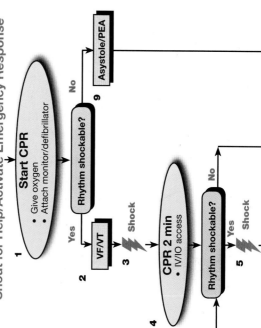

1
Start CPR
- Give oxygen
- Attach monitor/defibrillator

Rhythm shockable?

Yes — **2** VF/VT — **3** Shock

No — **9** Asystole/PEA

4 CPR 2 min
- IV/IO access

Rhythm shockable?

Yes — **5** Shock

No

Doses/Details

CPR Quality
- Push hard (≥2 inches [5 cm]) and fast (≥100/min) and allow complete chest recoil
- Minimize interruptions in compressions
- Avoid excessive ventilation
- Rotate compressor every 2 minutes
- If no advanced airway, 30:2 compression-ventilation ratio
- Quantitative waveform capnography
  – If $PETCO_2$ <10 mm Hg, attempt to improve CPR quality
- Intra-arterial pressure
  – If relaxation phase (diastolic) pressure <20 mm Hg, attempt to improve CPR quality

Return of Spontaneous Circulation (ROSC)
- Pulse and blood pressure
- Abrupt sustained increase in $PETCO_2$ (typically ≥40 mm Hg)
- Spontaneous arterial pressure waves with intra-arterial monitoring

Shock Energy
- **Biphasic:** Manufacturer recommendation (eg, initial dose of 120-200 J); if unknown, use maximum available.

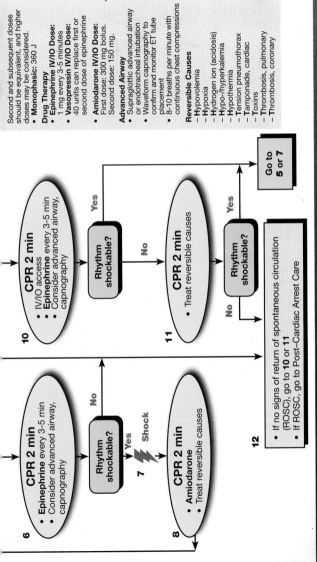

Second and subsequent doses should be equivalent, and higher doses may be considered.
• **Monophasic:** 360 J

Drug Therapy
• **Epinephrine IV/IO Dose:**
  1 mg every 3-5 minutes
• **Vasopressin IV/IO Dose:**
  40 units can replace first or second dose of epinephrine
• **Amiodarone IV/IO Dose:**
  First dose: 300 mg bolus.
  Second dose: 150 mg.

Advanced Airway
• Supraglottic advanced airway or endotracheal intubation
• Waveform capnography to confirm and monitor ET tube placement
• 8-10 breaths per minute with continuous chest compressions

Reversible Causes
— Hypovolemia
— Hypoxia
— Hydrogen ion (acidosis)
— Hypo-/hyperkalemia
— Hypothermia
— Tension pneumothorax
— Tamponade, cardiac
— Toxins
— Thrombosis, pulmonary
— Thrombosis, coronary

6
CPR 2 min
• Epinephrine every 3-5 min
• Consider advanced airway, capnography

Rhythm shockable?
No
Yes → ⚡ Shock **7**

8
CPR 2 min
• Treat reversible causes

10
CPR 2 min
• IV/IO access
• Epinephrine every 3-5 min
• Consider advanced airway, capnography

Rhythm shockable?
No
Yes → Go to 5 or 7

11
CPR 2 min
• Treat reversible causes

Rhythm shockable?
No
Yes → Go to 5 or 7

12
• If no signs of return of spontaneous circulation (ROSC), go to 10 or 11
• If ROSC, go to Post–Cardiac Arrest Care

6

Cardiac Arrest Circular Algorithm

Shout for Help/Activate Emergency Response

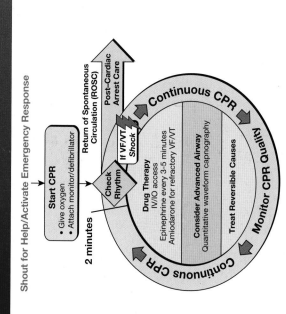

Start CPR
- Give oxygen
- Attach monitor/defibrillator

2 minutes

Check Rhythm

If VF/VT Shock

Return of Spontaneous Circulation (ROSC)

Post-Cardiac Arrest Care

Continuous CPR

Continuous CPR

Monitor CPR Quality

Drug Therapy
IV/IO access
Epinephrine every 3-5 minutes
Amiodarone for refractory VF/VT

Consider Advanced Airway
Quantitative waveform capnography

Treat Reversible Causes

Doses/Details

CPR Quality

- Push hard (≥2 inches [5 cm]) and fast (≥100/min) and allow complete chest recoil
- Minimize interruptions in compressions
- Avoid excessive ventilation
- Rotate compressor every 2 minutes
- If no advanced airway, 30:2 compression-ventilation ratio
- Quantitative waveform capnography
  - If $PETCO_2$ <10 mm Hg, attempt to improve CPR quality
- Intra-arterial pressure
  - If relaxation phase (diastolic) pressure <20 mm Hg, attempt to improve CPR quality

Return of Spontaneous Circulation (ROSC)

- Pulse and blood pressure
- Abrupt sustained increase in $PETCO_2$ (typically ≥40 mm Hg)
- Spontaneous arterial pressure waves with intra-arterial monitoring

Shock Energy

- **Biphasic:** Manufacturer recommendation (eg, initial dose of 120-200 J); if unknown, use maximum available. Second and subsequent doses should be equivalent, and higher doses may be considered.
- **Monophasic:** 360 J

Drug Therapy

- **Epinephrine IV/IO Dose:** 1 mg every 3-5 minutes
- **Vasopressin IV/IO Dose:** 40 units can replace first or second dose of epinephrine
- **Amiodarone IV/IO Dose:** First dose: 300 mg bolus. Second dose: 150 mg.

Advanced Airway

- Supraglottic advanced airway or endotracheal intubation
- Waveform capnography to confirm and monitor ET tube placement
- 8-10 breaths per minute with continuous chest compressions

Reversible Causes

- Hypovolemia
- Hypoxia
- Hydrogen ion (acidosis)
- Hypo-/hyperkalemia
- Hypothermia
- Tension pneumothorax
- Tamponade, cardiac
- Toxins
- Thrombosis, pulmonary
- Thrombosis, coronary

Immediate Post–Cardiac Arrest Care Algorithm

Doses/Details

Ventilation/Oxygenation
Avoid excessive ventilation.
Start at 10-12 breaths/min
and titrate to target $PETCO_2$
of 35-40 mm Hg.
When feasible, titrate FIO_2
to minimum necessary to
achieve Spo_2 ≥94%.

IV Bolus
1-2 L normal saline
or lactated Ringer's.
If inducing hypothermia,
may use 4°C fluid.

Epinephrine IV Infusion:
0.1-0.5 mcg/kg per minute
(in 70-kg adult: 7-35 mcg
per minute)

Return of Spontaneous Circulation (ROSC)

↓

Optimize ventilation and oxygenation
- Maintain oxygen saturation ≥94%
- Consider advanced airway and waveform capnography
- Do not hyperventilate

↓

**Treat hypotension
(SBP <90 mm Hg)**
- IV/IO bolus
- Vasopressor infusion
- Consider treatable
  causes
- 12-Lead ECG

Dopamine IV Infusion:
5-10 mcg/kg per minute

Norepinephrine IV Infusion:
0.1-0.5 mcg/kg per minute
(in 70-kg adult: 7-35 mcg per
minute)

Reversible Causes
– Hypovolemia
– Hypoxia
– Hydrogen ion (acidosis)
– Hypo-/hyperkalemia
– Hypothermia
– Tension pneumothorax
– Tamponade, cardiac
– Toxins
– Thrombosis, pulmonary
– Thrombosis, coronary

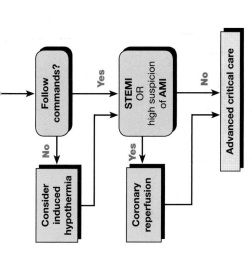

Bradycardia With a Pulse Algorithm

Assess appropriateness for clinical condition.
Heart rate typically <50/min if bradyarrhythmia.

Identify and treat underlying cause

- Maintain patent airway; assist breathing as necessary
- Oxygen (if hypoxemic)
- Cardiac monitor to identify rhythm; monitor blood pressure and oximetry
- IV access
- 12-Lead ECG if available; don't delay therapy

Persistent bradyarrhythmia causing:

- Hypotension?
- Acutely altered mental status?
- Signs of shock?
- Ischemic chest discomfort?
- Acute heart failure?

No → **Monitor and observe**

Yes

Doses/Details

Atropine IV Dose:
First dose: 0.5 mg bolus
Repeat every 3-5 minutes
Maximum: 3 mg

Dopamine IV Infusion:
2-10 mcg/kg per minute

Epinephrine IV Infusion:
2-10 mcg per minute

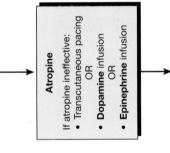

Atropine

If atropine ineffective:
- Transcutaneous pacing
  OR
- **Dopamine** infusion
  OR
- **Epinephrine** infusion

Consider:
- Expert consultation
- Transvenous pacing

Tachycardia With a Pulse Algorithm

Assess appropriateness for clinical condition.
Heart rate typically ≥150/min if tachyarrhythmia.

Identify and treat underlying cause

- Maintain patent airway; assist breathing as necessary
- Oxygen (if hypoxemic)
- Cardiac monitor to identify rhythm; monitor blood pressure and oximetry

Persistent tachyarrhythmia causing:

- Hypotension?
- Acutely altered mental status?
- Signs of shock?
- Ischemic chest discomfort?
- Acute heart failure?

No

Yes

Synchronized cardioversion

- Consider sedation
- If regular narrow complex, consider adenosine

Doses/Details

Synchronized Cardioversion

Initial recommended doses:

- Narrow regular: 50-100 J
- Narrow irregular:
  120-200 J biphasic or
  200 J monophasic
- Wide regular: 100 J
- Wide irregular: defibrillation dose (NOT synchronized)

Wide QRS?
≥0.12 second

Yes

- IV access and 12-lead ECG if available
- Consider adenosine only if regular and monomorphic
- Consider antiarrhythmic infusion
- Consider expert consultation

No

- IV access and 12-lead ECG if available
- Vagal maneuvers
- Adenosine (if regular)
- β-Blocker or calcium channel blocker
- Consider expert consultation

Adenosine IV Dose:
First dose: 6 mg rapid IV push; follow with NS flush.
Second dose: 12 mg if required.

Antiarrhythmic Infusions for Stable Wide-QRS Tachycardia

Procainamide IV Dose:
20-50 mg/min until arrhythmia suppressed, hypotension ensues, QRS duration increases >50%, or maximum dose 17 mg/kg given.
Maintenance infusion: 1-4 mg/min. Avoid if prolonged QT or CHF.

Amiodarone IV Dose:
First dose: 150 mg over 10 minutes. Repeat as needed if VT recurs. Follow by maintenance infusion of 1 mg/min for first 6 hours.

Sotalol IV Dose:
100 mg (1.5 mg/kg) over 5 minutes. Avoid if prolonged QT.

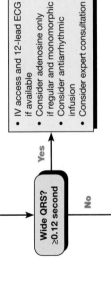

Relationship Between QT Interval and Heart Rate

Rhythm strips A and B demonstrate the requirement to evaluate the QT interval in light of the heart rate. Strip C depicts an ECG from a patient with a prolonged QT interval.

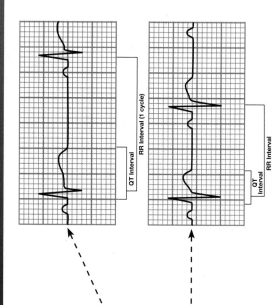

- *Strip A:* A bradycardic rhythm of 57/min has a QT interval of 0.4 second, which is less than the upper limit of normal for a rate of 57 (0.41 second for a man and 0.45 second for a woman), and a QT/R-R ratio of 38% (<40%).

- *Strip B:* A faster rate of 78/min has a shorter measured QT interval of 0.24 second (faster-shorter/slower-longer), which is less than the upper limit of normal for a rate of 78 (0.35 second for a man and 0.38 second for a woman), and a QT/R-R ratio of 33% (<40%).

- *Strip C:* Here the QT interval is prolonged at 0.45 second, exceeding the upper limit of normal for a rate of 80/min (0.34 second for a man and 0.37 second for a woman). The QT/R-R ratio of 59% is considerably above the 40% threshold. This strip is from a patient who took an overdose of a tricyclic antidepressant.

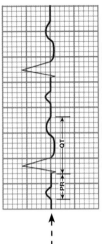

Prolonged QT interval: toxic drug effects

Parameter	Rhythm Strip A	Rhythm Strip B	Rhythm Strip C
Rate	57/min	78/min	80/min
R-R interval (cardiac cycle time)	1.04 seconds (26 × 1-mm boxes)	0.72 second (18 × 1-mm boxes)	0.76 second (19 × 1-mm boxes)
QT interval, measured	0.4 second (10 × 1-mm boxes)	0.24 second (6 × 1-mm boxes)	0.45 second (11 × 1-mm boxes)
QT$_c$ interval: QT interval corrected for heart rate (upper limit of normal QT interval range for a man or a woman from table on next page)	0.41 second (man) 0.45 second (woman)	0.35 second (man) 0.38 second (woman)	0.34 second (man) 0.37 second (woman)
QT/R-R ratio: QT interval divided by R-R interval	38% (0.4/1.04 = 0.384)	33% (0.24/0.72 = 0.333)	59% (0.45/0.76 = 0.592)

From Cummins RO, Graves JR. *ACLS Scenarios: Core Concepts for Case-Based Learning.* St Louis, MO: Mosby Lifeline; 1996. Figures modified with permission from Elsevier.

Maximum QT Interval (Upper Limits of Normal) for Men and Women Based on Heart Rate

Note the relationship between decreasing heart rate and increasing maximum QT interval. For normal heart rate range of 60 to 100 per minute (gray), the maximum QT intervals for men and women (light blue) are less than one half the R-R interval (marigold). Most people estimate QT and R-R intervals by counting the number of 1-mm boxes and then multiplying by 0.04 second. The third column was added to eliminate the need to multiply by 0.04.

Heart Rate (per minute)	R-R Interval (sec)	Upper Limits of Normal QT Interval (sec)	
(note decreasing)	Or "Cycle Time" (note increasing)	Men (note increasing)	Women (note increasing)
150	0.4	0.25	0.28
136	0.44	0.26	0.29
125	0.48	0.28	0.3
115	0.52	0.29	0.32
107	0.56	0.3	0.33
100	0.6	0.31	0.34
93	0.64	0.32	0.35
88	0.68	0.33	0.36

78	0.72	0.35	0.38
75	0.8	0.36	0.39
71	0.84	0.37	0.4
68	0.88	0.38	0.41
65	0.92	0.38	0.42
62	0.96	0.39	0.43
60	1	0.4	0.44
57	1.04	0.41	0.45
52	1.08	0.42	0.47
50	1.2	0.44	0.48

From Cummins RO, Graves JR. *ACLS Scenarios: Core Concepts for Case-Based Learning.* St Louis, MO: Mosby Lifeline; 1996.

Electrical Cardioversion Algorithm

Steps for Adult Defibrillation and Cardioversion

Using Manual Defibrillators (Monophasic or Biphasic)

Assess the rhythm. If VF or pulseless VT is present, continue chest compressions without interruptions during all steps until step 8.

Defibrillation (for VF and pulseless VT)

1. Turn on defibrillator. For biphasic defibrillators use manufacturer-specific energy if known. For monophasic defibrillators use 360 J. If unknown select the maximum energy available.
2. Set lead select switch to *paddles* (or *lead I, II, or III* if monitor leads are used).
3. Prepare adhesive pads (pads are preferred); if using paddles, apply appropriate conductive gel or paste. Be sure cables are attached to defibrillator.
4. Position defibrillation pads on patient's chest: one on the right anterior chest wall and one in the left axillary position. If paddles are used, apply firm pressure (about 15-25 pounds) when ready to deliver shock. If patient has an implanted pacemaker, position the pads so they are not directly over the device. Be sure that oxygen flow is not directed across the patient's chest.
5. Announce "Charging defibrillator!"
6. Press *charge* button on apex paddle or defibrillator controls.
7. When the defibrillator is fully charged, state firmly:
   "I am going to shock on three." Then count. "All clear!"
   (Chest compressions should continue until this announcement.)
8. After confirming all personnel are clear of the patient, press the *shock* button on the defibrillator or press the 2 paddle *discharge* buttons simultaneously.
9. Immediately after the shock is delivered, resume CPR beginning with compressions for 5 cycles (about 2 minutes), and then recheck rhythm. Interruption of CPR should be brief.

Tachycardia
With serious signs and symptoms related to the tachycardia

If ventricular rate is >150/min, prepare for **immediate cardioversion.** May give brief trial of medications based on specific arrhythmias. Immediate cardioversion is generally not needed if heart rate is ≤150/min.

Have available at bedside
- Oxygen saturation monitor
- Suction device
- IV line
- Intubation equipment

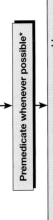

Premedicate whenever possible*

Synchronized cardioversion†‡

Atrial fibrillation§	120-200 J, increase in stepwise fashion (per manufacturer's recommendation)
Stable monomorphic VT‖	100 J, increase in stepwise fashion (per manufacturer's recommendation)
Other SVT, atrial flutter‖	50-100 J, increase in stepwise fashion (per manufacturer's recommendation)

Notes:

*Effective regimens have included a sedative (eg, **diazepam, midazolam, etomidate, methohexital, propofol**) with or without an analgesic agent (eg, **fentanyl, morphine**). Many experts recommend anesthesia if service is readily available.

†Note possible to resynchronize after each cardioversion.

‡If delays in synchronization occur and clinical condition is critical, go immediately to unsynchronized shocks.

§These doses are for biphasic waveforms. For monophasic waveforms, initial dose is 200 J for atrial fibrillation.

‖Recommended biphasic and monophasic doses are equivalent.

Cardioversion (for tachycardia with a pulse)

Assess the rhythm. If patient has a pulse but is unstable, proceed with cardioversion.

1-4. Follow steps for defibrillation above (except for energy dose).

5. Consider sedation.

6. Engage the *synchronization* mode by pressing the sync control button.

7. Look for markers on R waves indicating *sync* mode is operative. If necessary, adjust monitor gain until sync markers occur with each R wave.

8. Select appropriate energy level (see Electrical Cardioversion Algorithm on left).

9. Announce "Charging defibrillator!"

10. Press *charge* button on apex paddle or defibrillator controls.

11. When the defibrillator is fully charged, state firmly: "I am going to shock on three." Then count. "All clear!"

12. After confirming all personnel are clear of the patient, press the *discharge* buttons simultaneously on paddles or the *shock* button on the unit; hold paddles in place until shock is delivered.

13. Check the monitor. If tachycardia persists, increase the energy and prepare to cardiovert again.

14. Reset the *sync* mode after each synchronized cardioversion because most defibrillators default back to unsynchronized mode. This default allows an immediate shock if the cardioversion produces VF.

Therapy	Indications/Precautions	Adult Dosage
Cardioversion (Synchronized) Administered via adhesive defibrillation electrode pads or handheld paddles Place defibrillator/monitor in synchronized (sync) mode Sync mode delivers energy concurrent with the QRS	**Indications** • All unstable tachycardias (rate >150/min) with signs and symptoms related to tachycardia (acutely altered mental status, ischemic chest discomfort, acute heart failure, hypotension, or other signs of shock). • A brief trial of medications is an alternative first step for specific arrhythmias. **Precautions/Contraindications** • In critical conditions go to immediate unsynchronized shocks. • Urgent cardioversion is generally not needed if heart rate is ≤150/min. • Be sure oxygen is not flowing across patient's chest. Direct flow away from patient's chest and consider temporarily disconnecting bag or ventilation circuit from endotracheal tube during shock delivery. • Reactivation of sync mode is required after each attempted cardioversion (defibrillator/ cardioverter defaults to unsynchronized mode). • Prepare to defibrillate immediately if cardioversion causes VF.	**Technique** • Premedicate with sedatives whenever possible. • Engage **sync** mode before each attempt. • Look for sync markers on the R wave. • Clear all personnel from the patient before each shock. • For regular narrow-complex tachycardias, such as reentry SVT and atrial flutter, start with 50 J to 100 J. If initial dose fails, increase in stepwise fashion. • For irregular narrow-complex tachycardia consistent with atrial fibrillation, use 200 J initial monophasic shock, or 120 to 200 J initial biphasic shock, and then increase in stepwise fashion. • For regular wide complex tachycardia consistent with monomorphic VT, start with 100 J. If initial dose fails, increase in stepwise fashion. • Irregular wide complex tachycardia consistent with unstable polymorphic VT (irregular form and rate) should be treated with high-energy unsynchronized dose used for VF: 360 J monophasic waveform or biphasic device-specific defibrillation dose.

(continued)

Cardioversion (continued)

- Some defibrillators cannot deliver synchronized cardioversion unless the patient is also connected to monitor leads; in other defibrillators, ECG leads are incorporated into the defibrillation pads. Lead select switch may need to be on *lead I, II,* or *III* and not on *paddles*.
- Press *charge* button, *clear* the patient, and press both *shock* buttons simultaneously. Be prepared to perform CPR or defibrillation.

Transcutaneous Pacing

Generally external pacemakers allow adjustment of heart rate and current outputs

Indications

- Unstable bradycardia (<50/min) with signs and symptoms related to the bradycardia (hypotension, acutely altered mental status, signs of shock, ischemic chest discomfort, or acute heart failure) unresponsive to drug therapy.
- Be ready to pace in setting of AMI, as follows:
  - Markedly symptomatic sinus node dysfunction
  - Type II second-degree heart block
  - Third-degree heart block
  - New left, right, or alternating BBB or bifascicular block
- Symptomatic bradycardia with ventricular escape rhythms.
- Not recommended for agonal rhythms or cardiac arrest.

Precautions

- Conscious patients may require analgesia for discomfort.
- Avoid using carotid pulse to confirm mechanical capture. Electrical stimulation causes muscular jerking that may mimic carotid pulse.

Technique

- Position pacing electrodes on chest per package instructions.
- Turn pacer *on*.
- Set demand rate to approximately 80/min.
- Set current (mA) output as follows for bradycardia: increase current from minimum setting until consistent capture is achieved (characterized by a widening QRS and a broad T wave after each pacer spike).

Maternal Cardiac Arrest Algorithm

First Responder

- Activate maternal cardiac arrest team
- Document time of onset of maternal cardiac arrest
- Place the patient in the supine position
- Start chest compressions as per BLS algorithm but place hands slightly higher on sternum than usual

Subsequent Responders

Maternal Interventions
Treat per BLS and ACLS Algorithms

- Do not delay defibrillation
- Give typical ACLS drugs and doses
- Ventilate with 100% oxygen
- Monitor waveform capnography and CPR quality
- Provide post–cardiac arrest care as appropriate

Obstetric Interventions for Patient With an Obviously Gravid Uterus*

- Perform manual left uterine displacement (LUD)—displace uterus to the patient's left to relieve aortocaval compression
- Remove both internal and external fetal monitors if present

Maternal Modifications

- Start IV above the diaphragm
- Assess for hypovolemia and give fluid bolus when required
- Anticipate difficult airway; experienced provider preferred for advanced airway placement
- If patient receiving IV/IO magnesium prearrest, stop magnesium and give IV/IO calcium chloride 10 mL in 10% solution, or calcium gluconate 30 mL in 10% solution
- Continue all maternal resuscitative interventions (CPR, positioning, defibrillation, drugs, and fluids) during and after cesarean section

Obstetric and neonatal teams should immediately prepare for possible emergency cesarean section

- If no ROSC by 4 minutes of resuscitative efforts, consider performing immediate emergency cesarean section
- Aim for delivery within 5 minutes of onset of resuscitative efforts

*An obviously gravid uterus is a uterus that is deemed clinically to be sufficiently large to cause aortocaval compression

Search for and Treat Possible Contributing Factors (BEAU-CHOPS)

Bleeding/DIC
Embolism: coronary/pulmonary/amniotic fluid embolism
Anesthetic complications
Uterine atony
Cardiac disease (MI/ischemia/aortic dissection/cardiomyopathy)
Hypertension/preeclampsia/eclampsia
Other: differential diagnosis of standard ACLS guidelines
Placenta abruptio/previa
Sepsis

Suspected Stroke Algorithm

Identify signs and symptoms of possible stroke
Activate Emergency Response

Critical EMS assessments and actions
- Support ABCs; give **oxygen** if needed
- Perform prehospital stroke assessment
- Establish time of symptom onset (last normal)
- Triage to stroke center
- Alert hospital
- Check glucose if possible

Immediate general assessment and stabilization
- Assess ABCs, vital signs
- Provide **oxygen** if hypoxemic
- Obtain IV access and perform laboratory assessments
- Check glucose; treat if indicated
- Perform neurologic screening assessment
- Activate stroke team
- Order emergent CT scan or MRI of brain
- Obtain 12-lead ECG

Immediate neurologic assessment by stroke team or designee
- Review patient history
- Establish time of symptom onset or last known normal
- Perform neurologic examination (NIH Stroke Scale or Canadian Neurological Scale)

NINDS TIME GOALS

ED Arrival

10 min

ED Arrival

25 min

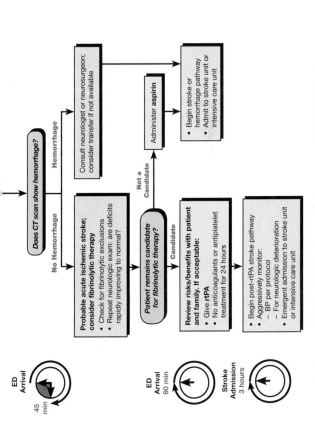

ED Arrival
45 min

Does CT scan show hemorrhage?

No Hemorrhage

Probable acute ischemic stroke; consider fibrinolytic therapy
• Check for fibrinolytic exclusions
• Repeat neurologic exam: are deficits rapidly improving to normal?

Hemorrhage

Consult neurologist or neurosurgeon; consider transfer if not available

Patient remains candidate for fibrinolytic therapy?

Not a Candidate

Administer **aspirin**

• Begin stroke or hemorrhage pathway
• Admit to stroke unit or intensive care unit

Candidate

ED Arrival
60 min

Review risks/benefits with patient and family. If acceptable:
• Give **rtPA**
• No anticoagulants or antiplatelet treatment for 24 hours

Stroke Admission
3 hours

• Begin post-rtPA stroke pathway
• Aggressively monitor:
  – BP per protocol
  – For neurologic deterioration
• Emergent admission to stroke unit or intensive care unit

16

The 8 D's of Stroke Care

The 8 D's of stroke care highlight the major steps in diagnosis and treatment of stroke and key points at which delays can occur:

Detection	Rapid recognition of stroke symptoms
Dispatch	Early activation and dispatch of emergency medical services (EMS) system by calling 911
Delivery	Rapid EMS identification, management, and transport
Door	Appropriate triage to stroke center
Data	Rapid triage, evaluation, and management within the ED
Decision	Stroke expertise and therapy selection
Drug	Fibrinolytic therapy, intra-arterial strategies
Disposition	Rapid admission to stroke unit, critical care unit

Modified from Demystifying recognition and management of stroke. *Currents in Emergency Cardiac Care.* 1996;7:8.

Out-of-Hospital Assessment of the Patient With Acute Stroke

- Perform initial assessment
  - Assess and support airway, breathing, and circulation as needed
  - Determine level of consciousness
  - Measure vital signs frequently
- Obtain relevant history
  - Identify time of symptom onset or last seen normal
  - Identify any seizure activity
  - Determine recent illness, injury, or surgery
- Perform physical examination
  - Conduct general medical examination
    - Cardiovascular abnormalities
  - Determine blood glucose level
  - Observe for signs of trauma
  - Conduct neurologic examination
    - Glasgow Coma Scale
    - Perform prehospital stroke screen (eg, Cincinnati Prehospital Stroke Scale, Los Angeles Prehospital Stroke Screen)
- Once possible stroke identified
  - Provide prearrival notification to receiving hospital of potential stroke patient
  - Triage to the nearest appropriate stroke hospital
  - Bring family member or transport witness if possible

Adult Stroke Assessment and General Management

The Cincinnati Prehospital Stroke Scale

Facial Droop (have the patient show teeth or smile):
- Normal—both sides of face move equally
- Abnormal—one side of face does not move as well as the other side

Arm Drift (patient closes eyes and extends both arms straight out, with palms up, for 10 seconds):
- Normal—both arms move the same or both arms do not move at all (other findings, such as pronator drift, may be helpful)
- Abnormal—one arm does not move or one arm drifts down compared with the other

Abnormal Speech (have the patient say "you can't teach an old dog new tricks"):
- Normal—patient uses correct words with no slurring
- Abnormal—patient slurs words, uses the wrong words, or is unable to speak

Interpretation: If any 1 of these 3 signs is abnormal, the probability of a stroke is 72%.

Left: normal. Right: stroke patient with facial droop (right side of face).

Modified from Kothari RU, Pancioli A, Liu T, Brott T, Broderick J. Cincinnati Prehospital Stroke Scale: reproducibility and validity. *Ann Emerg Med.* 1999;33:373-378. With permission from Elsevier.

Glasgow Coma Scale*

Score (maximum = 15)

Eye opening

Spontaneous	4
In response to speech	3
In response to pain	2
None	1

Best verbal response

Oriented conversation	5
Confused conversation	4
Inappropriate words	3
Incomprehensible sounds	2
None	1

Best motor response

Obeys	6
Localizes	5
Withdraws	4
Abnormal flexion	3
Abnormal extension	2
None	1

Interpretation:

Score 14 to 15: Mild dysfunction
Score 11 to 13: Moderate to severe dysfunction
Score ≤10: Severe dysfunction

*Teasdale G, Jennett B. Assessment of coma and impaired consciousness: a practical scale. *Lancet.* 1974;2(7872):81-84.

General Management of the Acute Stroke Patient

1. **Intravenous fluids:** Avoid D₅W and excessive fluid loading.

2. **Blood sugar:** Determine immediately. Bolus of 50% dextrose if hypoglycemic; insulin if serum glucose >185 mg/dL (threshold varies; check institution/system protocol).

3. **Cardiac monitoring:** During first 24 hours.

4. **Oxygen:** Pulse oximetry. Supplement for oxyhemoglobin saturation <94%.

5. **Acetaminophen:** If febrile.

6. **NPO:** Perform swallowing assessment.

Use of IV rtPA for Acute Ischemic Stroke: Inclusion and Exclusion Characteristics

Patients Who Could Be Treated With rtPA Within 3 *Hours* From Symptom Onset[*]

Inclusion Criteria

- Diagnosis of ischemic stroke causing measurable neurologic deficit
- Onset of symptoms <3 hours before beginning treatment
- Age ≥18 years

Exclusion Criteria

- Head trauma or prior stroke in previous 3 months
- Symptoms suggest subarachnoid hemorrhage
- Arterial puncture at noncompressible site in previous 7 days
- History of previous intracranial hemorrhage
- Elevated blood pressure (systolic >185 mm Hg or diastolic >110 mm Hg)
- Evidence of active bleeding on examination
- Acute bleeding diathesis, including but not limited to
  - Platelet count <100 000/mm^3
  - Heparin received within 48 hours, resulting in aPTT >upper limit of normal
  - Current use of anticoagulant with INR >1.7 or PT >15 seconds

Exclusion Criteria (*continued*)

- Blood glucose concentration <50 mg/dL (2.7 mmol/L)
- CT demonstrates multilobar infarction (hypodensity >⅓ cerebral hemisphere)

Relative Exclusion Criteria

Recent experience suggests that under some circumstances—with careful consideration and weighing of risk to benefit—patients may receive fibrinolytic therapy despite 1 or more relative contraindications. Consider risk to benefit of rtPA administration carefully if any one of these relative contraindications is present:

- Only minor or rapidly improving stroke symptoms (clearing spontaneously)
- Seizure at onset with postictal residual neurologic impairments
- Major surgery or serious trauma within previous 14 days
- Recent gastrointestinal or urinary tract hemorrhage (within previous 21 days)
- Recent acute myocardial infarction (within previous 3 months)

Abbreviations: aPTT, activated partial thromboplastin time; INR, international normalized ratio; PT, prothrombin time; rtPA, recombinant tissue plasminogen activator.

*Adams HP Jr, del Zoppo G, Alberts MJ, Bhatt DL, Brass L, Furlan A, Grubb RL, Higashida RT, Jauch EC, Kidwell C, Lyden PD, Morgenstern LB, Qureshi AI, Rosenwasser RH, Scott PA, Wijdicks EFM. Guidelines for the early management of adults with ischemic stroke: a guideline from the American Heart Association/American Stroke Association Stroke Council, Clinical Cardiology Council, Cardiovascular Radiology and Intervention Council, and the Atherosclerotic Peripheral Vascular Disease and Quality of Care Outcomes in Research Interdisciplinary Working Groups. *Stroke*. 2007;38:1655-1711.

Use of IV rtPA for Acute Ischemic Stroke: Additional Inclusion and Exclusion Characteristics

Patients Who Could Be Treated With rtPA From 3 to 4.5 Hours From Symptom Onset[†]

Inclusion Criteria

- Diagnosis of ischemic stroke causing measurable neurologic deficit
- Onset of symptoms 3 to 4.5 hours before beginning treatment

Exclusion Criteria

- Age >80 years
- Severe stroke (NIHSS >25)
- Taking an oral anticoagulant regardless of INR
- History of both diabetes and prior ischemic stroke

Notes

- The checklist includes some US FDA–approved indications and contraindications for administration of rtPA for acute ischemic stroke. Recent AHA/ASA guideline revisions may differ slightly from FDA criteria. A physician with expertise in acute stroke care may modify this list.
- Onset time is either witnessed or last known normal.

Notes *(continued)*

- In patients without recent use of oral anticoagulants or heparin, treatment with rtPA can be initiated before availability of coagulation study results but should be discontinued if INR is >1.7 or PT is elevated by local laboratory standards.
- In patients without history of thrombocytopenia, treatment with rtPA can be initiated before availability of platelet count but should be discontinued if platelet count is <100 000/mm^3.

Abbreviations: FDA, Food and Drug Administration; INR, international normalized ratio; NIHSS, National Institutes of Health Stroke Scale; PT, prothrombin time; rtPA, recombinant tissue plasminogen activator.

†del Zoppo GJ, Saver JL, Jauch EC, Adams HP Jr; on behalf of the American Heart Association Stroke Council. Expansion of the time window for treatment of acute ischemic stroke with intravenous tissue plasminogen activator: a science advisory from the American Heart Association/American Stroke Association. *Stroke.* 2009;40:2945-2948.

Stroke: Treatment of Hypertension

Potential Approaches to Arterial Hypertension in Acute Ischemic Stroke Patients Who Are Potential Candidates for Acute Reperfusion Therapy*

Patient otherwise eligible for acute reperfusion therapy except that blood pressure is >185/110 mm Hg:

- Labetalol 10-20 mg IV over 1-2 minutes, may repeat × 1, or
- Nicardipine IV 5 mg per hour, titrate up by 2.5 mg per hour every 5-15 minutes, maximum 15 mg per hour; when desired blood pressure is reached, lower to 3 mg per hour, or
- Other agents (hydralazine, enalaprilat, etc) may be considered when appropriate

If blood pressure is not maintained at or below 185/110 mm Hg, do not administer rtPA.

Management of blood pressure during and after rtPA or other acute reperfusion therapy:

Monitor blood pressure every 15 minutes for 2 hours from the start of rtPA therapy, then every 30 minutes for 6 hours, and then every hour for 16 hours.

If systolic blood pressure 180-230 mm Hg or diastolic blood pressure 105-120 mm Hg:

- Labetalol 10 mg IV followed by continuous IV infusion 2-8 mg per minute, or
- Nicardipine IV 5 mg per hour, titrate up to desired effect by 2.5 mg per hour every 5-15 minutes, maximum 15 mg per hour

If blood pressure not controlled or diastolic blood pressure >140 mm Hg, consider sodium nitroprusside.

Approach to Arterial Hypertension in Acute Ischemic Stroke Patients Who Are *Not* Potential Candidates for Acute Reperfusion Therapy*

Consider lowering blood pressure in patients with acute ischemic stroke if systolic blood pressure >220 mm Hg or diastolic blood pressure >120 mm Hg.

Consider blood pressure reduction as indicated for other concomitant organ system injury:

- Acute myocardial infarction
- Congestive heart failure
- Acute aortic dissection

A reasonable target is to lower blood pressure by 15% to 25% within the first day.

*Adams HP Jr, del Zoppo G, Alberts MJ, Bhatt DL, Brass L, Furlan A, Grubb RL, Higashida RT, Jauch EC, Kidwell C, Lyden PD, Morgenstern LB, Qureshi AI, Rosenwasser RH, Scott PA, Wijdicks EFM. Guidelines for the early management of adults with ischemic stroke: a guideline from the American Heart Association/American Stroke Association Stroke Council, Clinical Cardiology Council, Cardiovascular Radiology and Intervention Council, and the Atherosclerotic Peripheral Vascular Disease and Quality of Care Outcomes in Research Interdisciplinary Working Groups. *Stroke*. 2007;38:1655-1711.

Acute Coronary Syndromes Algorithm

Symptoms suggestive of ischemia or infarction

↓

EMS assessment and care and hospital preparation
- Monitor, support ABCs. Be prepared to provide CPR and defibrillation
- Administer aspirin and consider oxygen, nitroglycerin, and morphine if needed
- Obtain 12-lead ECG; if ST elevation:
  - Notify receiving hospital with transmission or interpretation; note time of onset and first medical contact
  - Notified hospital should mobilize hospital resources to respond to STEMI
- If considering prehospital fibrinolysis, use fibrinolytic checklist

↓

Concurrent ED assessment (<10 minutes)
- Check vital signs; evaluate oxygen saturation
- Establish IV access
- Perform brief, targeted history, physical exam
- Review/complete fibrinolytic checklist; check contraindications
- Obtain initial cardiac marker levels, initial electrolyte and coagulation studies
- Obtain portable chest x-ray (<30 minutes)

Immediate ED general treatment
- If O₂ sat <94%, start **oxygen** at 4 L/min, titrate
- **Aspirin** 160 to 325 mg (if not given by EMS)
- **Nitroglycerin** sublingual or spray
- **Morphine** IV if discomfort not relieved by nitroglycerin

↓

ECG interpretation

↓

| **ST elevation or new or presumably new LBBB; strongly suspicious for injury** ST-elevation MI (STEMI) | **ST depression or dynamic T-wave inversion; strongly suspicious for ischemia** High-risk unstable angina/ non–ST-elevation MI (UA/NSTEMI) | **Normal or nondiagnostic changes in ST segment or T wave** Low-/intermediate-risk ACS |

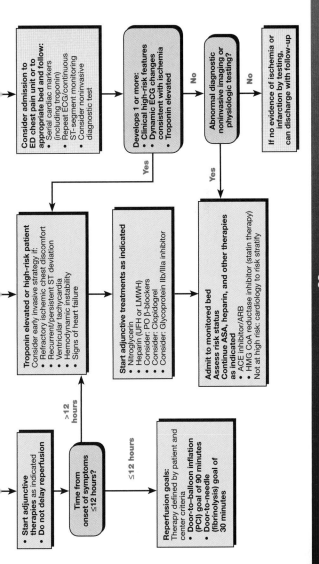

Consider admission to ED chest pain unit or to appropriate bed and follow:
- Serial cardiac markers (including troponin)
- Repeat ECG/continuous ST-segment monitoring
- Consider noninvasive diagnostic test

Develops 1 or more:
- Clinical high-risk features
- Dynamic ECG changes consistent with ischemia
- Troponin elevated

Yes →

No

Abnormal diagnostic noninvasive imaging or physiologic testing?

Yes →

No

If no evidence of ischemia or infarction by testing, can discharge with follow-up

Troponin elevated or high-risk patient
Consider early invasive strategy if:
- Refractory ischemic chest discomfort
- Recurrent/persistent ST deviation
- Ventricular tachycardia
- Hemodynamic instability
- Signs of heart failure

Start adjunctive treatments as indicated
- Nitroglycerin
- Heparin (UFH or LMWH)
- Consider: PO β-blockers
- Consider: Clopidogrel
- Consider: Glycoprotein IIb/IIIa inhibitor

Admit to monitored bed
Assess risk status
Continue ASA, heparin, and other therapies as indicated
- ACE inhibitor/ARB
- HMG CoA reductase inhibitor (statin therapy)
Not at high risk: cardiology to risk stratify

Start adjunctive therapies as indicated
- Do not delay reperfusion

Time from onset of symptoms ≤12 hours?

>12 hours ↑

≤12 hours ↓

Reperfusion goals:
Therapy defined by patient and center criteria
- Door-to-balloon inflation (PCI) goal of 90 minutes
- Door-to-needle (fibrinolysis) goal of 30 minutes

22

Likelihood That Signs and Symptoms Represent an ACS Secondary to CAD

Feature	High Likelihood *Any of the following:*	Intermediate Likelihood *Absence of high-likelihood features and presence of any of the following:*	Low Likelihood *Absence of high- or intermediate-likelihood features but may have the following:*
History	Chest or left arm pain or discomfort as chief symptom reproducing prior documented angina Known history of CAD, including MI	Chest or left arm pain or discomfort as chief symptom Age >70 years Male sex Diabetes mellitus	Probable ischemic symptoms in absence of any intermediate-likelihood characteristics Recent cocaine use
Examination	Transient MR murmur, hypotension, diaphoresis, pulmonary edema, or rales	Extracardiac vascular disease	Chest discomfort reproduced by palpation

ECG	New or presumably new transient ST-segment deviation (≥1 mm) or T-wave inversion in mutiple precordial leads	Fixed Q waves ST depression 0.5 to 1 mm or T-wave inversion >1 mm	T-wave flattening or inversion <1 mm in leads with dominant R waves Normal ECG
Cardiac markers	Elevated cardiac TnI, TnT, or CK-MB	Normal	Normal

Abbreviations: CAD, coronary artery disease; CK-MB, MB fraction of creatine kinase; ECG, electrocardiogram; MI, myocardial infarction; MR, mitral regurgitation; TnI, troponin I; TnT, troponin T.

Reproduced from 2007 Focused Update of the ACC/AHA/SCAI 2005 Guideline Update for Percutaneous Coronary Intervention: a report of the American College of Cardiology/American Heart Association Task Force on Practice Guidelines. *Circulation.* 2008;117:261–295. Modified from Braunwald E, Mark DB, Jones RH, et al. *Unstable Angina: Diagnosis and Management. Clinical Practice Guideline No. 10.* Rockville, MD: Agency for Health Care Policy and Research and the National Heart, Lung, and Blood Institute, Public Health Service, US Department of Health and Human Services; 1994. AHCPR publication 94-0602.

Acute Coronary Syndromes: Fibrinolytic Checklist for STEMI*

Step 1

Has patient experienced chest discomfort for greater than 15 minutes and less than 12 hours?

YES → NO → **STOP**

Does ECG show STEMI or new or presumably new LBBB?

YES → NO →

Step 2

Are there contraindications to fibrinolysis?
If ANY one of the following is checked YES, fibrinolysis MAY be contraindicated.

Systolic BP >180 to 200 mm Hg or diastolic BP >100 to 110 mm Hg   ○ YES   ○ NO

Right vs left arm systolic BP difference >15 mm Hg   ○ YES   ○ NO

History of structural central nervous system disease   ○ YES   ○ NO

Significant closed head/facial trauma within the previous 3 weeks   ○ YES   ○ NO

Stroke >3 hours or <3 months   ○ YES   ○ NO

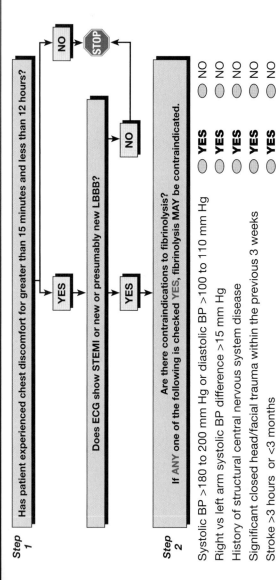

Recent (within 2-4 weeks) major trauma, surgery (including laser eye surgery), GI/GU bleed   ○ **YES**   ○ NO

Any history of intracranial hemorrhage   ○ **YES**   ○ NO

Bleeding, clotting problem, or blood thinners   ○ **YES**   ○ NO

Pregnant female   ○ **YES**   ○ NO

Serious systemic disease (eg, advanced cancer, severe liver or kidney disease)   ○ **YES**   ○ NO

Step 3	Is patient at high risk? If ANY one of the following is checked YES, consider transfer to PCI facility.

Heart rate ≥100/min AND systolic BP <100 mm Hg   ○ **YES**   ○ NO

Pulmonary edema (rales)   ○ **YES**   ○ NO

Signs of shock (cool, clammy)   ○ **YES**   ○ NO

Contraindications to fibrinolytic therapy   ○ **YES†**   ○ NO

Required CPR   ○ **YES**   ○ NO

24

*Contraindications for fibrinolytic use in STEMI consistent with "Thrombolytic Therapy and Balloon Angioplasty in Acute ST Elevation Myocardial Infarction (STEMI)" at Agency for Healthcare Research and Quality National Guideline Clearinghouse (www.Guidelines.gov).

†Consider transport to primary PCI facility as destination hospital.

Acute Coronary Syndromes: Fibrinolytic Agents*

Alteplase, Recombinant (rtPA)	Streptokinase

Recommended total dose is based on patient's weight.
• Accelerated infusion (1.5 hours)
  – Give 15 mg IV bolus.
  – Then 0.75 mg/kg over next 30 minutes (not to exceed 50 mg).
  – Then 0.5 mg/kg over 60 minutes (not to exceed 35 mg).
  – Maximum total dose: 100 mg.
	1.5 million units in a 1-hour infusion.

Reteplase, Recombinant

- Give first 10 unit IV bolus over 2 minutes.
- 30 minutes later give second 10 unit IV bolus over 2 minutes. (Give NS flush before and after each bolus.)

Tenecteplase

- Bolus, weight adjusted
  - <60 kg: Give 30 mg.
  - 60-69 kg: Give 35 mg.
  - 70-79 kg: Give 40 mg.
  - 80-89 kg: Give 45 mg.
  - ≥90 kg: Give 50 mg.
- Administer single IV bolus over 5 seconds.
- Incompatible with dextrose solutions.

*See Advanced Cardiovascular Life Support Drugs section for complete details.

Immediate General Treatment

- Oxygen
- Aspirin
- Nitroglycerin
- Morphine (if unresponsive to nitrates)

Oxygen

If oxygen saturation <94% or evidence of respiratory distress: 4 L/min per nasal cannula; titrate to maintain $Sao_2 \geq 94\%$.

- **Uncomplicated MI:** Reasonable to use until stabilization. Probably not helpful beyond 6 hours.
- **Complicated MI** (for overt pulmonary congestion): Administer supplementary O_2 at 4 L/min by nasal cannula; titrate as needed (maintain $Sao_2 \geq 94\%$).

Aspirin

For all patients with ACS unless true aspirin allergy exists (then consider clopidogrel), in either out-of-hospital or ED setting.

Cautions and Contraindications

- Active peptic ulcer disease (use rectal suppositories).
- History of true aspirin allergy.
- Bleeding disorders, severe hepatic disease.

Recommended Dosing

- Give 160 to 325 mg non-enteric-coated orally, crushed or chewed (may use rectal suppository if cannot give by mouth).

Nitroglycerin

Indicated for patients with ischemic-type chest pain.

Cautions and Contraindications

- The use of nitrates in patients with hypotension (SBP <90 mm Hg or ≥30 mm Hg below baseline), extreme bradycardia (<50/min), or tachycardia (>100/min) in the absence of heart failure is contraindicated.

- Administer nitrates with extreme caution, if at all, to patients with inferior wall MI and suspected right ventricular involvement, because these patients require adequate RV preload. (Obtain right-sided ECG leads to assist in diagnosing RV infarct.)

- Contraindicated in patients who have used phosphodiesterase inhibitor for erectile dysfunction (eg, sildenafil or vardenafil within 24 hours; tadalafil within 48 hours).

Recommended Dosing

- SL: 0.3 to 0.4 mg, repeat × 2 at 3- to 5-minute intervals OR
- Spray: 1 or 2 sprays, may repeat × 2 at 3- to 5-minute intervals OR
- IV: 12.5 to 25 mcg bolus (if no SL or spray given); then 10 mcg per minute infusion, titrated (increased at a rate of 10 mcg per minute every 3 to 5 minutes until symptom response or target arterial pressure is achieved). Ceiling dose of 200 mcg per minute commonly used.

Morphine

Indicated for patients with ischemic pain not relieved by nitroglycerin.

Cautions and Contraindications

- Do not use in patients with hypotension.
- Use cautiously in patients with suspected hypovolemia.
- A large observational registry demonstrated an association between morphine use and mortality in patients with UA/NSTEMI. The clinical significance of this observation is not clear; however, the AHA/ACC has changed the recommendation for morphine use in this patient population to Class IIa.

Recommended Dosing: STEMI

Give 2 to 4 mg IV; may give additional doses of 2 to 8 mg IV at 5- to 15-minute intervals.

Recommended Dosing: UA/NSTEMI

Give 1 to 5 mg IV only if symptoms not relieved by nitrates or if symptoms recur.

Acute Coronary Syndromes: Triage

Triage and Assessment of Cardiac Risk in the Emergency Department
Stratifying Patients With Possible or Probable ACS in the ED

- **Protocols must be in place to stratify** chest pain patients by risk of ACS. **The 12-lead ECG is central to ED triage of patients with ACS.** Stratify patients into one of the following subgroups (also see below):

  1. **ST-segment elevation or new LBBB:** High specificity for evolving STEMI; assess reperfusion eligibility.

  2. **ST-segment depression:** Consistent with/strongly suggestive of ischemia; defines a high-risk subset of patients with UA/NSTEMI. Especially important if there are new or dynamic ECG changes. Clinical correlation is necessary to interpret completely.

  3. **Nondiagnostic or normal ECG:** Further assessment usually needed; evaluation protocols should include repeat ECG or continuous ST-segment monitoring and serial cardiac markers. Myocardial imaging or 2D echocardiogram may be useful during medical observation in selected patients. Noninvasive testing (ie, stress test/cardiac imaging) should be considered if ECG and serial markers remain normal.

- **Clinicians should carefully consider the diagnosis of ACS even in the absence of typical chest discomfort. Consider ACS in patients with**
  - Anginal equivalent symptoms, such as dyspnea (LV dysfunction), palpitations, presyncope, and syncope (ischemic ventricular arrhythmias)
  - Atypical left precordial pain or complaint of indigestion or dyspepsia
  - Atypical pain in the elderly, women, and persons with diabetes

- **Continually consider other causes of chest pain:** aortic dissection, pericarditis/myocarditis, pulmonary embolus

- **Fibrinolytic therapy:** Administer as soon as possible; optimal door-to-drug time of ≤30 minutes

- **PCI:** Identify reperfusion candidates promptly and achieve balloon inflation as soon as possible with primary PCI; optimal door-to-balloon inflation time of ≤90 minutes

Emergency Department Triage Recommendations

- **Symptoms and signs indicating need for immediate assessment and ECG within 10 minutes of presentation**
  - Chest or epigastric discomfort, nontraumatic in origin with components typical for ischemia or MI
  - Central substernal compression or crushing pain; pressure, tightness, heaviness, cramping, burning, aching sensation; unexplained indigestion, belching, epigastric pain; radiating pain in neck, jaws, shoulders, back, or one or both arms
  - Associated dyspnea, nausea or vomiting, diaphoresis
  - Palpitations, irregular pulse, or suspected arrhythmia

- **For all patients with ischemic-type chest pain**
  - Provide supplementary oxygen (until stable, for saturation <94% or respiratory distress), IV access, and continuous ECG monitoring
  - Prompt interpretation of 12-lead ECG by physician responsible for ACS triage

- **For all patients with STEMI**
  - Initiate protocol for reperfusion therapy (fibrinolytics or PCI)
  - Rule out contraindications and assess risk-benefit ratio
  - Consider primary PCI if available or if patient is ineligible for fibrinolytics
  - PCI (or CABG if indicated) is the preferred reperfusion treatment for patients presenting in cardiogenic shock

- **For all patients with moderate- to high-risk non–ST-segment elevation ACS and STEMI**
  - Prompt aspirin (160 to 325 mg) unless given in past 24 hours
  - Clopidogrel (300 mg loading dose)
  - Oral β-blockers for all patients without contraindications, when stable; IV β-blockers for patients with hypertension or tachyarrhythmias without contraindications; routine IV β-blockers are otherwise not recommended

- **IV nitroglycerin for initial 24 to 48 hours only in patients with AMI and CHF, large anterior infarction, recurrent or persistent ischemia, or hypertension**

Relationship of 12-Lead ECG to Coronary Artery Anatomy

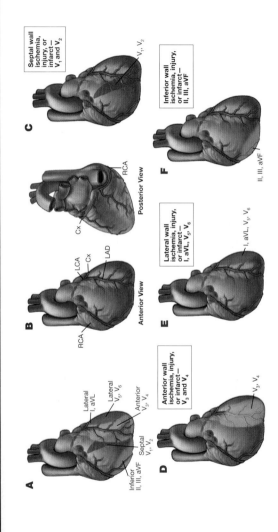

A — Lateral I, aVL; Lateral V_5, V_6; Anterior V_3, V_4; Septal V_1, V_2; Inferior II, III, aVF

B — Anterior View: RCA, LCA, Cx, LAD; Posterior View: Cx, RCA

C — Septal wall ischemia, injury, or infarct — V_1 and V_2

D — Anterior wall ischemia, injury, or infarct — V_3 and V_4

E — Lateral wall ischemia, injury, or infarct — I, aVL, V_5, V_6

F — Inferior wall ischemia, injury, or infarct — II, III, aVF

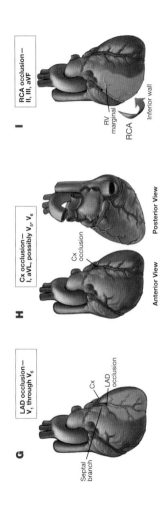

G | LAD occlusion— V_1 through V_6

Septal branch
LAD occlusion
Cx

H | Cx occlusion— I, aVL, possibly V_5, V_6

Anterior View

Posterior View

Cx occlusion

I | RCA occlusion— II, III, aVF

RV marginal
RCA
Inferior wall

I lateral	aVR	V_1 septal	V_4 anterior
II inferior	aVL lateral	V_2 septal	V_5 lateral
III inferior	aVF inferior	V_3 anterior	V_6 lateral

Localizing ischemia, injury, or infarct using the 12-lead ECG: relationship to coronary artery anatomy.

How to Measure ST-Segment Deviation

Inferior MI
ST segment has no low point (it is coved or concave).

Anterior MI

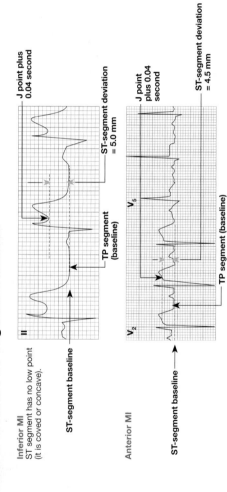

ECG Lead Changes Due to Injury or Infarct With Coronary Artery, Anatomical Area of Damage, and Associated Complications

Leads With ECG Changes	Injury/Infarct-Related Artery	Area of Damage	Associated Complications
V_1-V_2	LCA: LAD-septal branch	Septum, His bundle, bundle branches	Infranodal block and BBBs
V_3-V_4	LCA: LAD-diagonal branch	Anterior wall LV	LV dysfunction, CHF, BBBs, complete heart block, PVCs
V_5-V_6 plus I and aVL	LCA: circumflex branch	High lateral wall LV	LV dysfunction, AV nodal block in some
II, III, aVF	RCA: posterior descending branch	Inferior wall LV, posterior wall LV	Hypotension, sensitivity to nitroglycerin and morphine sulfate
V_4R (II, III, aVF)	RCA: proximal branches	RV, inferior wall LV, posterior wall LV	Hypotension, supranodal and AV-nodal blocks, atrial fibrillation/flutter, PACs, adverse medical reactions
V_1 through V_4 (marked depression)	Either LCA-circumflex or RCA-posterior descending branch	Posterior wall LV	LV dysfunction

Abbreviations: AV, atrioventricular; BBB, bundle branch block; CHF, congestive heart failure; ECG, electrocardiographic; LAD, left anterior descending artery; LCA, left coronary artery; LV, left ventricle (left ventricular); PAC, premature atrial complex; PVC, premature ventricular complex; RCA, right coronary artery; RV, right ventricle.

Acute ST-Segment Elevation
Potential Adjunctive Therapies (Do Not Delay Reperfusion to Administer)
β-Blockers

Rationale: Block sympathetic nervous system stimulation of heart rate and vasoconstriction. Decrease myocardial oxygen consumption and increase myocardial salvage in area of infarct and can reduce incidence of ventricular ectopy and fibrillation.

Caution: Early aggressive β-blockade poses a net hazard in hemodynamically unstable patients and should be avoided. IV β-blockers should not be administered to STEMI or UA/NSTEMI patients who have any of the following:

- Moderate to severe LV failure and pulmonary edema
- Bradycardia (<60/min)
- Hypotension (SBP <100 mm Hg)
- Signs of poor peripheral perfusion
- Second-degree or third-degree heart block
- Reactive airway disease

STEMI and UA/NSTEMI Recommendations

- Oral β-blocker therapy should be initiated in the first 24 hours for patients who do not have any of the contraindications listed above.

- It is reasonable to administer an intravenous β-blocker at the time of presentation to STEMI patients who are hypertensive or have tachyarrhythmias and who do not have any of the contraindications listed above.

- Patients with early contraindications within the first 24 hours of STEMI should be reevaluated for candidacy for β-blocker therapy as secondary prevention. Patients with moderate or severe LV failure should receive β-blocker therapy as secondary prevention with a gradual titration scheme.

Heparin for Acute Coronary Syndromes

- **STEMI–Fibrinolytic Adjunct:** Anticoagulant therapy for a minimum of 48 hours and preferably the duration of hospitalization, up to 8 days. Regimens other than unfractionated heparin (UFH) are recommended if anticoagulant therapy is given for more than 48 hours. Recommended regimens include

  – UFH: Initial bolus 60 units/kg (maximum 4000 units) followed by intravenous infusion of 12 units/kg per hour (maximum 1000 units per hour) initially adjusted to maintain the aPTT at 50 to 70 seconds (duration of treatment 48 hours or until angiography).

  – Enoxaparin (if serum creatinine <2.5 mg/dL in men and 2 mg/dL in women): If age <75 years, an initial bolus of 30 mg IV is followed 15 minutes later by subcutaneous injections 1 mg/kg every 12 hours (maximum 100 mg for first 2 doses only). If age ≥75 years, the initial bolus is eliminated, and subcutaneous dose is reduced to 0.75 mg/kg every 12 hours (maximum 75 mg for first 2 doses only). Regardless of age, if serum creatinine during course of treatment is estimated to be <30 mL/min (using Cockroft-Gault formula), the subcutaneous regimen is 1 mg/kg every 24 hours.

  – Patients initially treated with enoxaparin should not be switched to UFH and vice versa because of increased risk of bleeding.

  – Fondaparinux (provided serum creatinine <3 mg/dL and creatinine clearance ≥30 mL/min): Initial dose 2.5 mg IV; subsequent subcutaneous injections 2.5 mg every 24 hours. Maintenance dosing should be continued for duration of hospitalization, up to 8 days.

- **UA/NSTEMI: For patients at high to intermediate risk, anticoagulant therapy should be added to antiplatelet therapy. Initial invasive strategy:**

  – UFH: Use same as above.

  – Enoxaparin: Maintenance dose: If creatinine clearance ≥30 mL/min, give 1 mg/kg subcutaneously every 12 hours. If creatinine clearance <30 mL/min, give 1 mg/kg once every 24 hours. Patients initially treated with enoxaparin should not be switched to UFH and vice versa because of increased risk of bleeding.

  – Fondaparinux: 2.5 mg subcutaneously every 24 hours. Contraindicated if creatinine clearance <30 mL/min.

  – Bivalirudin: 0.1 mg/kg bolus; maintenance 0.25 mg/kg per hour infusion.

ST-Segment Elevation or New or Presumably New LBBB: Evaluation for Reperfusion

Step 1: Assess time and risk

- Time since onset of symptoms
- Risk of STEMI (TIMI Risk Score for STEMI)
- Risk of fibrinolysis
- Time required to transport to skilled percutaneous coronary intervention (PCI) catheterization suite (first medical contact/door-to-balloon time)

Step 2: Select reperfusion (fibrinolysis or invasive) strategy

Note: If presentation ≤3 hours from symptom onset and no delay for PCI, then no preference for either strategy.

Fibrinolysis is generally preferred if:	An invasive strategy is generally preferred if:
• Early presentation (≤3 hours from symptom onset)	• Late presentation (symptom onset >3 hours ago)
• Invasive strategy is not an option (eg, lack of access to skilled PCI facility or difficult vascular access) or would be delayed • Medical contact–to-balloon or door-to-balloon time >90 min	• Skilled PCI facility available with surgical backup • Medical contact–to-balloon or door-to-balloon time <90 min
• No contraindications to fibrinolysis	• Contraindications to fibrinolysis, including increased risk of bleeding and ICH
	• High risk from STEMI (eg, presenting in shock or conges-tive heart failure)
	• Diagnosis of STEMI is in doubt

Evaluate for Primary PCI

Can restore vessel patency and normal flow with >90% success in experienced high-volume centers with experienced providers

Primary PCI is most effective for the following:

- In cardiogenic shock patients (<75 years old) if performed ≤18 hours from onset of shock and ≤36 hours from onset of ST-elevation infarction. However, up to 40% of shock patients require coronary artery bypass grafting (CABG) for optimal management.
- In selected patients >75 years old with STEMI and cardiogenic shock.
- In patients with indications for reperfusion but with a contraindication to fibrinolytic therapy.

Best results achieved at PCI centers with these characteristics:

- Centers with high volume (>200 PCI procedures per year; at least 36 are primary PCI)
- Experienced operator (>75 PCI procedures per year) with technical skill
- Balloon dilation <90 minutes from initial medical contact or ED presentation
- Achievement of normal flow rate (TIMI grade 3) in >90% of cases without emergency CABG, stroke, or death
  - At least 50% resolution of maximal ST-segment elevation (microvascular reperfusion)

Evaluate for Fibrinolytic Therapy: Assess Eligibility and Risk-Benefit Ratio

Early treatment (door-to-drug time ≤30 minutes) can limit infarct size, preserve LV function, and reduce mortality.

- Maximum myocardial salvage occurs with early fibrinolytic administration, although a reduction in mortality may still be observed up to 12 hours from onset of continuous persistent symptoms.
- Normal flow achieved in 54% of patients treated with accelerated rtPA, in 33% of patients treated with streptokinase and heparin.

Most effective in the following patients:

- Early presentation
- Larger infarction
- Low risk of intracerebral hemorrhage

Benefits with age and delayed presentation:

- Patients >75 years of age have increased risk of cerebral hemorrhage but absolute benefit similar to younger patients.
- Generally not recommended if presentation 12 to 24 hours after symptom onset.

May be harmful:

- ST-Segment depression (may be harmful and should not be used unless true posterior MI present)
- Patients >24 hours after onset of pain
- Number of risk factors (age [≥65 years], low body weight [<70 kg], initial hypertension [≥180/110 mm Hg]) predicts frequency of hemorrhagic stroke: no risk factors = 0.25%; 3 risk factors = 2.5%

Fibrinolytic Therapy

Contraindications for fibrinolytic use in STEMI consistent with ACC/AHA 2007 Focused Update*

Absolute Contraindications

- Any prior intracranial hemorrhage
- Known structural cerebral vascular lesion (eg, arteriovenous malformation)
- Known malignant intracranial neoplasm (primary or metastatic)
- Ischemic stroke within 3 months EXCEPT acute ischemic stroke within 3 hours
- Suspected aortic dissection
- Active bleeding or bleeding diathesis (excluding menses)
- Significant closed head trauma or facial trauma within 3 months

Relative Contraindications

- History of chronic, severe, poorly controlled hypertension
- Severe uncontrolled hypertension on presentation (SBP >180 mm Hg or DBP >110 mm Hg)†
- History of prior ischemic stroke >3 months, dementia, or known intracranial pathology not covered in contraindications
- Traumatic or prolonged (>10 minutes) CPR or major surgery (<3 weeks)
- Recent (within 2 to 4 weeks) internal bleeding
- Noncompressible vascular punctures
- For streptokinase/anistreplase: prior exposure (>5 days ago) or prior allergic reaction to these agents
- Pregnancy
- Active peptic ulcer
- Current use of anticoagulants: the higher the INR, the higher the risk of bleeding

*Viewed as advisory for clinical decision making and may not be all-inclusive or definitive.

†Could be an absolute contraindication in low-risk patients with myocardial infarction.

Update: Universal Definition of AMI

- Detection of a rise and fall of cardiac biomarkers (preferably troponin) with at least 1 value above the 99th percentile of the upper reference limit (URL) and at least 1 of the following:
  - Symptoms of ischemia
  - ECG changes of ischemia: ST-T changes or new LBBB
  - Development of pathologic Q waves
  - Imaging evidence of loss of viable myocardium or new regional wall-motion abnormality

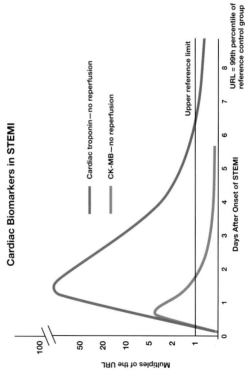

Cardiac Biomarkers in STEMI

Modified from ACC/AHA 2007 Guidelines for the Management of Patients With Unstable Angina/Non-ST-Elevation Myocardial Infarction: Executive Summary. *Circulation.* 2007;116:827; and Shapiro BP, Jaffe AS. Cardiac biomarkers. In: Murphy JG, Lloyd MA, eds. *Mayo Clinic Cardiology: Concise Textbook.* 3rd ed. Rochester, MN: Mayo Clinic Scientific Press and Informa Healthcare USA; 2007:773-779.

Cardiac Troponins

- Troponin I and troponin T are cardiac-specific structural proteins not normally detected in serum. Patients with increased troponin levels have increased thrombus burden and microvascular embolization.
- Preferred biomarker for diagnosis of MI. Increased sensitivity compared with CK-MB. Elevation above 99th percentile of mean population value is diagnostic.
- Detect minimal myocardial damage in patients with UA/NSTEMI.
  - 30% of patients without ST-segment elevation who would otherwise be diagnosed with UA have small amounts of myocardial damage when troponin assays are used (eg, CK-MB negative).
  - These patients are at increased risk for major adverse cardiac events and may benefit from new therapies such as GP IIb/IIIa inhibitors compared with patients who lack elevations in these cardiac-specific markers.
- Useful in risk stratification because patients with elevated serum troponin concentrations are at increased risk for subsequent nonfatal MI and sudden cardiac death.
  - Can also be used to detect reinfarction.
  - Remain elevated for 7-14 days after infarct.

CK-MB

- Present in skeletal muscle and serum, less specific than troponin.
- Marker for reinfarction and noninvasive assessment of reperfusion.

TIMI Risk Score for Patients With Unstable Angina and Non–ST-Segment Elevation MI: Predictor Variables

Predictor Variable	Point Value of Variable	Definition
Age ≥65 years	1	
≥3 risk factors for CAD	1	**Risk factors:** • Family history of CAD • Hypertension • Hypercholesterolemia • Diabetes • Current smoker
Aspirin use in last 7 days	1	
Recent, severe symptoms of angina	1	≥2 anginal events in last 24 hours
Elevated cardiac markers	1	CK-MB or cardiac-specific troponin level

| ST deviation ≥0.5 mm | 1 | ST depression ≥0.5 mm is significant; transient ST elevation ≥0.5 mm for <20 minutes is treated as ST-segment depression and is high risk; ST elevation >1 mm for more than 20 minutes places these patients in the STEMI treatment category. |
| Prior coronary artery stenosis ≥50% | 1 | Risk predictor remains valid even if this information is unknown. |

Calculated TIMI Risk Score	Risk of ≥1 Primary End Point* in ≤14 Days	Risk Status
0 or 1	5%	Low
2	8%	
3	13%	Intermediate
4	20%	
5	26%	High

*Primary end points: death, new or recurrent MI, or need for urgent revascularization.

Antman EM, Cohen M, Bernink PJLM, McCabe CH, Horacek T, Papuchis G, Mautner B, Corbalan R, Radley D, Braunwald E. The TIMI risk score for unstable angina/non-ST elevation MI: a method for prognostication and therapeutic decision making. *JAMA*. 2000;284:835-842.

Risk Stratification and Treatment Strategies for Patients With UA/NSTEMI

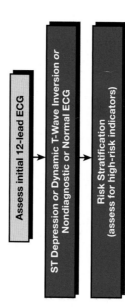

Risk Stratification Algorithm for chest discomfort patients with ST depression, dynamic T-wave inversions, nondiagnostic or normal ECG

Review
(at presentation and during observation)
- History
- Physical examination
- ECG
- Cardiac markers (troponin T or I; CK-MB)

Assess initial 12-lead ECG

ST Depression or Dynamic T-Wave Inversion or Nondiagnostic or Normal ECG

Risk Stratification
(assess for high-risk indicators)

TIMI Risk Score Factors

History:
- ☐ Age ≥65 years
- ☐ ≥3 risk factors for CAD
- ☐ Prior coronary artery stenosis ≥50%
- ☐ Aspirin use in past 7 days
- ☐ Recent, severe symptoms of angina

ECG:
- ☐ ST deviation ≥0.5 mm

Cardiac markers:
- ☐ Elevated cardiac markers

Review for ACC/AHA High-Risk Indicators
(in addition to the TIMI risk factors)

History:	☐ High (≥5) or Intermediate (3 or 4) TIMI risk score* ☐ PCI or prior CABG within 6 months
Physical Examination:	☐ Recurrent angina/ischemia with CHF symptoms, an S_3 gallop, pulmonary edema, worsening rales, or new or worsening mitral regurgitation
ECG and Cardiac Markers:	☐ Hemodynamic or electrical instability (ischemic VT) ☐ Elevated cardiac markers
Evaluation:	☐ High-risk findings on noninvasive stress testing ☐ Depressed LV systolic function (eg, EF <0.40 on noninvasive study) *TIMI risk score should be derived by experienced physicians. Application to all patients with chest discomfort is not indicated.

Does patient stratify as *high* or *intermediate* risk by 1 or more of the following:

☐ ST deviation? (original or subsequent ECG)
☐ TIMI risk score ≥5?
☐ TIMI risk score 3 or 4?

☐ Cardiac markers elevated?
☐ Age ≥75?
☐ Unstable angina (UA)?
☐ ACC/AHA high-risk indicator?

◀── **YES**   **NO** ──▶ **Low Risk: Conservative Strategy†**

High-Intermediate Risk: Invasive Strategy

†No benefit for early invasive strategy in low-risk women (may be excess risk with invasive strategy).

Acute Coronary Syndromes:
Treatment Recommendations for UA/NSTEMI

Glycoprotein IIb/IIIa Inhibitors
Recommendations

Actions

- Inhibit the integrin GP IIb/IIIa receptor in the platelet membrane.
- Inhibit final common pathway to activation of platelet aggregation.

Clinical trials

- While these drugs are often used as an adjunct to PCI, there are insufficient data to support the routine use of GP IIb/IIIa inhibitors in patients with suspected STEMI or UA/NSTEMI ACS in the prehospital or ED settings.

Available approved agents

- **Abciximab (ReoPro):** murine monoclonal antibody to the GP IIb/IIIa receptor.
- **Eptifibatide (Integrilin):** small-molecule cyclical heptapeptide that binds to the receptor; short half-life.
  - Contraindicated in renal dialysis patients.
- **Tirofiban (Aggrastat):** small-molecule nonpeptide, also with short half-life.

Thienopyridines (also called ADP Antagonists)
Recommendations

Clopidogrel

In patients <75 years of age with non–ST-segment elevation ACS and STEMI, regardless of approach to management, a loading dose of clopidogrel 300 to 600 mg is recommended.

- In patients for whom CABG is planned, clopidogrel should be withheld for at least 5 days unless the urgency for revascularization outweighs the risk of excess bleeding.
- In patients receiving any stent during PCI for ACS, clopidogrel 75 mg daily should be given for at least 12 months.
- For UA/NSTEMI patients treated medically, clopidogrel (75 mg/day orally) should be prescribed for at least 1 month and ideally for up to 1 year.
- Clopidogrel is indicated for patients unable to take aspirin.

Prasugrel

Prasugrel (60 mg oral loading dose) may be substituted for clopidogrel after angiography in patients found to have UA/NSTEMI ACS or STEMI who are more than 12 hours past symptom onset before planned PCI.

- Not recommended for STEMI patients managed with fibrinolysis or for UA/NSTEMI patients before angiography.
- In patients who are not at high risk for bleeding, administration of prasugrel (60 mg oral loading dose) before angiography in patients found to have STEMI ≤12 hours after the initial symptoms may be substituted for administration of clopidogrel.
- In patients for whom CABG is planned, prasugrel should be withheld for at least 7 days unless the urgency for revascularization outweighs the risk of excess bleeding.
- In patients receiving any stent during PCI for ACS, prasugrel 10 mg daily should be given for at least 12 months.

Ticagrelor

Ticagrelor is an alternative to clopidogrel for patients found to have NSTEMI or STEMI managed with early invasive strategy.

Communication With Family

Conveying News of a Sudden Death to Family Members

- Before talking to the family, obtain as much information as possible about the patient and the circumstances surrounding the death. Be ready to refer to the patient by name.

- Call the family if they have not been notified. Explain that their loved one has been admitted to the emergency department or critical care unit and that the situation is serious. If possible, family members should be told of the death in person, not over the telephone.

- When family members arrive, ask someone to take them to a private area. Walk in, introduce yourself, and sit down. Address the closest relative. Maintain eye contact and position yourself at the same level as family members (ie, sitting or standing).

- Enlist the aid of a social worker or a member of the clergy if possible.

- Briefly describe the circumstances leading to the death. Summarize the sequence of events. Avoid euphemisms such as "he's passed on," "she's no longer with us," or "he's left us." Instead use the words "death," "dying," or "dead."

- Allow time for family members to process the information. Make eye contact and touch. Convey your feelings with a simple phrase such as "You have my (our) sincere sympathy."

- Determine the patient's suitability for and wishes about tissue donation (use driver's license and patient records). Discuss with the family if possible.

- Allow as much time as necessary for questions and discussion. Review the events several times if needed.

- Allow family members the opportunity to see the patient. Prepare the family for what they will see. If equipment is still connected to the patient, tell the family. Equipment must be left in place for coroner's cases or when an autopsy is performed.

- Determine in advance what happens next and who will sign the death certificate. Physicians may impose burdens on staff and family if they fail to understand policies about death certification and disposition of the body.

- Offer to contact the patient's attending or family physician and to be available if there are further questions. Arrange for follow-up and continued support during the grieving period.

Family Presence During Resuscitation

According to surveys in the United States and the United Kingdom, most family members state that they would like to be present during the attempted resuscitation of a loved one. Parents and care providers of chronically ill patients are often knowledgeable about and comfortable with medical equipment and emergency procedures. Even family members with no medical background report that it is comforting to be at the side of a loved one and say goodbye during the final moments of life. Family members often do not ask if they can be present, but healthcare providers should offer the opportunity whenever possible. Ideally, a designated support person should remain with the family during the resuscitation to answer questions, clarify information, and comfort the family.

Relatives and friends present during resuscitation of a loved one report fewer incidences of posttraumatic avoidance behaviors, fewer grieving symptoms, and less intrusive imagery.

When family members are present during resuscitative efforts, sensitivity is heightened among resuscitation team members. A team member who is knowledgeable about resuscitation practices should be available to answer questions, provide comfort, and help the family during the resuscitation. Even when the resuscitation outcome is not optimal, families feel comforted to know they can be present to say goodbye, give comfort to their dying loved one, and begin the grieving process.

Advanced Cardiovascular Life Support Drugs

Administration Notes

Peripheral Intravenous (IV):	Resuscitation drugs administered via peripheral IV catheter should be followed by bolus of 20 mL IV fluid to move drug into central circulation. Then elevate extremity for 10 to 20 seconds.
Intraosseous (IO):	ACLS drugs that can be administered by IV route can be administered by IO route.
Endotracheal:	IV/IO administration is preferred because it provides more reliable drug delivery and pharmacologic effect. Drugs that can be administered by endotracheal route are noted in the table below. Optimal endotracheal doses have not been established. Medication delivered via endotracheal tube should be diluted in sterile water or NS to a volume of 5 to 10 mL. Provide several positive-pressure breaths after medication is instilled.

Drug/Therapy	Indications/Precautions	Adult Dosage
ACE Inhibitors (Angiotensin-Converting Enzyme Inhibitors)	**Indications** • ACE inhibitors reduce mortality and improve LV dysfunction in post-AMI patients. They help prevent adverse LV remodeling, delay progression of heart failure, and decrease sudden death and recurrent MI. • An ACE inhibitor should be administered orally within the first 24 hours after onset of AMI symptoms and continued long term if tolerated. • Clinical heart failure without hypotension in patients not responding to digitalis or diuretics. • Clinical signs of AMI with LV dysfunction. • LV ejection fraction <40%.	**Approach:** ACE inhibitor therapy should start with low-dose oral administration (with possible IV doses for some preparations) and increase steadily to achieve a full dose within 24 to 48 hours. An angiotensin receptor blocker (ARB) should be administered to patients intolerant of ACE inhibitors.

(continued)

Enalapril

Captopril

Lisinopril

Ramipril

Precautions/Contraindications for All ACE Inhibitors

- *Contraindicated* in pregnancy (may cause fetal injury or death).
- Contraindicated in angioedema.
- Hypersensitivity to ACE inhibitors.
- Reduce dose in renal failure (creatinine >2.5 mg/dL in men, >2 mg/dL in women). Avoid in bilateral renal artery stenosis.
- Serum potassium >5 mEq/L.
- Do not give if patient is hypotensive (SBP <100 mm Hg or >30 mm Hg below baseline) or volume depleted.
- Generally not started in ED; after reperfusion therapy has been completed and blood pressure has stabilized, start within 24 hours.

Enalapril (IV = Enalaprilat)
- **PO:** Start with a single dose of 2.5 mg. Titrate to 20 mg PO BID.
- **IV:** 1.25 mg IV initial dose over 5 minutes, then 1.25 to 5 mg IV every 6 hours. IV form is contraindicated in STEMI (risk of hypotension).

Captopril, AMI Dose
- Start with a single dose of 6.25 mg PO.
- Advance to 25 mg TID and then to 50 mg TID as tolerated.

Lisinopril, AMI Dose
- 5 mg within 24 hours of onset of symptoms, then
  - 5 mg given after 24 hours, then
  - 10 mg given after 48 hours, then
  - 10 mg once daily

Ramipril
- Start with a single dose of 2.5 mg PO. Titrate to 5 mg PO BID as tolerated.

Advanced Cardiovascular Life Support Drugs

Drug/Therapy	Indications/Precautions	Adult Dosage
Adenosine	**Indications** • First drug for most forms of stable narrow-complex SVT. Effective in terminating those due to reentry involving AV node or sinus node. • May consider for unstable narrow-complex reentry tachycardia while preparations are made for cardioversion. • Regular and monomorphic wide-complex tachycardia, thought to be or previously defined to be reentry SVT. • Does *not* convert atrial fibrillation, atrial flutter, or VT. • Diagnostic maneuver: stable narrow-complex SVT. **Precautions/Contraindications** • Contraindicated in poison/drug-induced tachycardia or second- or third-degree heart block. • Transient side effects include flushing, chest pain or tightness, brief periods of asystole or bradycardia, ventricular ectopy. • Less effective (larger doses may be required) in patients taking theophylline or caffeine. • Reduce initial dose to 3 mg in patients receiving dipyridamole or carbamazepine, in heart transplant patients, or if given by central venous access. • If administered for irregular, polymorphic wide-complex tachycardia/VT, may cause deterioration (including hypotension). • Transient periods of sinus bradycardia and ventricular ectopy are common after termination of SVT. • Safe and effective in pregnancy.	**IV Rapid Push** • Place patient in mild reverse Trendelenburg position before administration of drug. • Initial bolus of 6 mg given *rapidly* over 1 to 3 seconds followed by NS bolus of 20 mL; then elevate the extremity. • A second dose (12 mg) can be given in 1 to 2 minutes if needed. **Injection Technique** • Record rhythm strip during administration. • Draw up adenosine dose and flush in 2 separate syringes. • Attach both syringes to the IV injection port closest to patient. • Clamp IV tubing above injection port. • Push IV adenosine *as quickly as possible* (1 to 3 seconds). • While maintaining pressure on adenosine plunger, push NS flush *as rapidly as possible* after adenosine. • Unclamp IV tubing.

Adenosine Diphosphate (ADP) Antagonists (Thienopyridines)

Indications

Adjunctive antiplatelet therapy for acute coronary syndrome (ACS) patients.

Precautions/Contraindications

- Do not administer to patients with active pathologic bleeding (eg, peptic ulcer). Use with caution in patients with risk of bleeding.
- **Prasugrel is contraindicated in patients with a history of TIA or stroke; use with caution in patients ≥75 years old or <60 kg due to increased risk of fatal and intracranial bleeding and uncertain benefit.**
- Use with caution in the presence of hepatic impairment.
- **When CABG is planned, withhold ADP antagonists for 5 (for clopidogrel) or 7 (for prasugrel) days before CABG unless need for revascularization outweighs the risk of excess bleeding.**

Note: Combinations of loading and maintenance doses of different ADP antagonists (clopidogrel, prasugrel, and ticagrelor) are **not** recommended.

Clopidogrel (Plavix)
75 mg and 300 mg tabs available

(continued)

Clopidogrel

- For STEMI or moderate- to high-risk non-ST elevation ACS, including patients receiving fibrinolysis.
- Limited evidence in patients ≥75 years old.
- Substitute for aspirin if patient is unable to take aspirin.

→

Clopidogrel

- STEMI or moderate- to high-risk UA/non-ST-segment elevation ACS patient <75 years old: Administer loading dose of 300 to 600 mg orally followed by maintenance dose of 75 mg orally daily; full effects will not develop for several days.
- ED patients with suspected ACS unable to take aspirin: loading dose 300 mg.

Advanced Cardiovascular Life Support Drugs

Drug/Therapy	Indications/Precautions	Adult Dosage
Prasugrel (Effient) 5 mg and 10 mg tabs available	**Prasugrel** • May be substituted for clopidogrel after angiography in patients with NSTEMI or STEMI who are not at high risk for bleeding. • Not recommended for STEMI patients managed with fibrinolysis or for NSTEMI patients before angiography. • No data to support use in ED or prehospital setting.	**Prasugrel** • STEMI or UA/NSTEMI patient <75 years old managed with PCI: Administer loading dose of 60 mg PO followed by maintenance dose of 10 mg PO daily; full effects will not develop for several days. • Consider dose reduction to 5 mg PO daily in patients weighing <60 kg.
Ticagrelor	**Ticagrelor** • May be administered to patients with NSTEMI or STEMI who are treated with early invasive strategy.	

Amiodarone

Amiodarone is a complex drug with effects on sodium, potassium, and calcium channels as well as α- and β-adrenergic blocking properties. Patients must be hospitalized while the loading doses of amiodarone are administered. Amiodarone should be prescribed only by physicians who are experienced in the treatment of life-threatening arrhythmias, are thoroughly familiar with amiodarone's risks and benefits, and have access to laboratory facilities capable of adequately monitoring the effectiveness and side effects of amiodarone treatment.

Indications

Because its use is associated with toxicity, amiodarone is indicated for use in patients with life-threatening arrhythmias when administered with appropriate monitoring:

- VF/pulseless VT unresponsive to shock delivery, CPR, and a vasopressor.
- Recurrent, hemodynamically unstable VT.

With expert consultation amiodarone may be used for treatment of some atrial and ventricular arrhythmias.

Caution: Multiple complex drug interactions

VF/VT Cardiac Arrest Unresponsive to CPR, Shock, and Vasopressor

First dose: 300 mg IV/IO push.

Second dose (if needed): 150 mg IV/IO push.

Life-Threatening Arrhythmias

Maximum cumulative dose: 2.2 g IV over 24 hours. May be administered as follows:

- **Rapid infusion:** 150 mg IV over first 10 minutes (15 mg per minute). May repeat rapid infusion (150 mg IV) every 10 minutes as needed.
- **Slow infusion:** 360 mg IV over 6 hours (1 mg per minute).
- **Maintenance infusion:** 540 mg IV over 18 hours (0.5 mg per minute).

Precautions

- Rapid infusion may lead to hypotension.
- With multiple dosing, cumulative doses >2.2 g over 24 hours are associated with significant hypotension in clinical trials.
- Do not administer with other drugs that prolong QT interval (eg, procainamide).
- Terminal elimination is extremely long (half-life lasts up to 40 days).

Advanced Cardiovascular Life Support Drugs

Drug/Therapy	Indications/Precautions	Adult Dosage
Amrinone (See *Inamrinone*)		
Aspirin	**Indications** • Administer to all patients with ACS, particularly reperfusion candidates, unless hypersensitive to aspirin. • Blocks formation of thromboxane A_2, which causes platelets to aggregate and arteries to constrict. This reduces overall ACS mortality, reinfarction, and nonfatal stroke. • Any person with symptoms ("pressure," "heavy weight," "squeezing," "crushing") suggestive of ischemic pain. **Precautions/Contraindications** • Relatively contraindicated in patients with active ulcer disease or asthma. • Contraindicated in patients with known hypersensitivity to aspirin.	• 160 mg to 325 mg non–enteric-coated tablet as soon as possible (chewing is preferable). • May use rectal suppository (300 mg) for patients who cannot take orally.

Atropine Sulfate

Can be given via
endotracheal tube

Indications

- First drug for symptomatic sinus bradycardia.
- May be beneficial in presence of AV nodal block or ventricular asystole. **Will not be effective for infranodal (Mobitz type II) block.**
- Routine use during PEA or asystole is unlikely to have a therapeutic benefit.
- Organophosphate (eg, nerve agent) poisoning: extremely large doses may be needed.

Precautions

- Use with caution in presence of myocardial ischemia and hypoxia. Increases myocardial oxygen demand.
- Avoid in hypothermic bradycardia.
- Will not be effective for infranodal (type II) AV block and new third-degree block with wide QRS complexes. (In these patients may cause paradoxical slowing. Be prepared to pace or give catecholamines.)
- Doses of atropine <0.5 mg may result in paradoxical slowing of heart rate.

Bradycardia (With or Without ACS)

- 0.5 mg IV every 3 to 5 minutes as needed, not to exceed total dose of 0.04 mg/kg (total 3 mg).
- Use shorter dosing interval (3 minutes) and higher doses in severe clinical conditions.

Organophosphate Poisoning

Extremely large doses (2 to 4 mg or higher) may be needed.

41

Advanced Cardiovascular Life Support Drugs

Drug/Therapy	Indications/Precautions	Adult Dosage
β-Blockers Metoprolol Tartrate	**Indications (Apply to all β-blockers)** • Administer to all patients with suspected myocardial infarction and unstable angina in the absence of contraindication. These are effective antianginal agents and can reduce incidence of VF. • Useful as an adjunctive agent with fibrinolytic therapy. May reduce nonfatal reinfarction and recurrent ischemia.	**Metoprolol Tartrate (AMI Regimen)** • Initial IV dose: 5 mg slow IV at 5-minute intervals to a total of 15 mg. • Begin oral regimen to follow IV dose with 50 mg PO; titrate to effect.
Atenolol	• To convert to normal sinus rhythm or to slow ventricular response (or both) in supraventricular tachyarrhythmias (reentry SVT, atrial fibrillation, or atrial flutter). β-Blockers are second-line agents after adenosine. • To reduce myocardial ischemia and damage in AMI patients with elevated heart rate, blood pressure, or both.	**Atenolol (AMI Regimen)** • 5 mg IV over 5 minutes. • Wait 10 minutes, then give second dose of 5 mg IV over 5 minutes. • In 10 minutes, if tolerated well, begin oral regimen with 50 mg PO; titrate to effect.
Propranolol	• Labetalol recommended for emergency antihypertensive therapy for hemorrhagic and acute ischemic stroke. **Precautions/Contraindications (Apply to all β-blockers unless noted)** • Early aggressive β-blockade may be hazardous in hemodynamically unstable patients.	**Propranolol (for SVT)** • 0.5 to 1 mg over 1 minute, repeated as needed to a total dose of 0.1 mg/kg.

(continued)

Esmolol

- Do not give to patients with STEMI if any of the following are present:
  - Signs of heart failure.
  - Low cardiac output.
  - Increased risk for cardiogenic shock.
- Relative contraindications include PR interval >0.24 second, second- or third-degree heart block, active asthma, reactive airway disease, severe bradycardia, SBP <100 mm Hg.
- Concurrent IV administration with IV calcium channel blocking agents like verapamil or diltiazem can cause severe hypotension and bradycardia/heart block.
- Monitor cardiac and pulmonary status during administration.
- Propranolol is contraindicated and other β-blockers relatively contraindicated in cocaine-induced ACS.

Calcium Chloride

10% solution is 100 mg/mL

Indications

- Known or suspected hyperkalemia (eg, renal failure).
- Ionized hypocalcemia (eg, after multiple blood transfusions).
- As an antidote for toxic effects (hypotension and arrhythmias) from calcium channel blocker overdose or β-blocker overdose.

Precautions

- Do not use routinely in cardiac arrest.
- Do not mix with sodium bicarbonate.

Esmolol

- 0.5 mg/kg (500 mcg/kg) over 1 minute, followed by 0.05 mg/kg (50 mcg/kg) per minute infusion; maximum: 0.3 mg/kg (300 mcg/kg) per minute.
- If inadequate response after 5 minutes, may repeat 0.5 mg/kg (500 mcg/kg) bolus and then titrate infusion up to 0.2 mg/kg (200 mcg/kg) per minute. Higher doses unlikely to be beneficial.
- Has a short half-life (2 to 9 minutes).

Labetalol

- 10 mL IV push over 1 to 2 minutes.
- May repeat or double every 10 minutes to a maximum dose of 150 mg, or give initial dose as a bolus, then start infusion at 2 to 8 mg per minute.

Typical Dose

- 500 mg to 1000 mg (5 to 10 mL of a 10% solution) IV for hyperkalemia and calcium channel blocker overdose. May be repeated as needed.
- *Note:* Comparable dose of 10% calcium gluconate is 15 to 30 mL.

Labetalol

Advanced Cardiovascular Life Support Drugs

Drug/Therapy	Indications/Precautions	Adult Dosage
Clopidogrel (See *ADP Antagonists*)		
Digoxin-Specific Antibody Therapy Digibind (38 mg) or DigiFab (40 mg) (each vial binds about 0.5 mg digoxin)	**Indications** Digoxin toxicity with the following: • Life-threatening arrhythmias. • Shock or congestive heart failure. • Hyperkalemia (potassium level >5 mEq/L). • Steady-state serum levels >10 to 15 ng/mL for symptomatic patients. **Precautions** • Serum digoxin levels rise after digoxin antibody therapy and should not be used to guide continuing therapy.	**Chronic Intoxication** 3 to 5 vials may be effective. **Acute Overdose** • IV dose varies according to amount of digoxin ingested. See ACLS Toxicology. • Average dose is 10 vials; may require up to 20 vials. • See package insert for details.

Digoxin

0.25 mg/mL or
0.1 mg/mL supplied in
1 or 2 mL ampule
(totals = 0.1 to 0.5 mg)

Indications (may be of limited use)

- To slow ventricular response in atrial fibrillation or atrial flutter.
- Alternative drug for reentry SVT.

Precautions

- Toxic effects are common and are frequently associated with serious arrhythmias.
- Avoid electrical cardioversion if patient is receiving digoxin unless condition is life-threatening; use lower dose (10 to 20 J).

IV Administration

- Loading doses: 0.004 to 0.006 mg/kg (4 to 6 mcg/kg) initially over 5 minutes. Second and third boluses of 0.002 to 0.003 mg/kg (2 to 3 mcg/kg) to follow at 4- to 8-hour intervals (total loading dose 8 to 12 mcg/kg divided over 8 to 16 hours).
- Check digoxin levels no sooner than 4 hours after IV dose; no sooner than 6 hours after oral dose.
- Monitor heart rate and ECG.
- Maintenance dose is affected by body mass and renal function.
- *Caution:* Amiodarone interaction. Reduce digoxin dose by 50% when used with amiodarone.

Advanced Cardiovascular Life Support Drugs

Drug/Therapy	Indications/Precautions	Adult Dosage
Diltiazem	**Indications** • To control ventricular rate in atrial fibrillation and atrial flutter. May terminate reentrant arrhythmias that require AV nodal conduction for their continuation. • Use after adenosine to treat refractory reentry SVT in patients with narrow QRS complex and adequate blood pressure. **Precautions** • Do not use calcium channel blockers for wide-QRS tachycardias of uncertain origin or for poison/drug-induced tachycardia. • Avoid calcium channel blockers in patients with Wolff-Parkinson-White syndrome plus rapid atrial fibrillation or flutter, in patients with sick sinus syndrome, or in patients with AV block without a pacemaker. • *Caution:* Blood pressure may drop from peripheral vasodilation (greater drop with verapamil than with diltiazem).	**Acute Rate Control** • 15 to 20 mg (0.25 mg/kg) IV over 2 minutes. • May give another IV dose in 15 minutes at 20 to 25 mg (0.35 mg/kg) over 2 minutes. **Maintenance Infusion** 5 to 15 mg per hour, titrated to physiologically appropriate heart rate (can dilute in D_5W or NS).

(continued)

Diltiazem
(continued)

- Avoid in patients receiving oral β-blockers.
- Concurrent IV administration with IV β-blockers can cause severe hypotension and AV block.

Dobutamine

IV infusion

Indications

- Consider for pump problems (congestive heart failure, pulmonary congestion) with SBP of 70 to 100 mm Hg and *no* signs of shock.

Precautions/Contraindications

- **Contraindication:** Suspected or known poison/drug-induced shock.
- Avoid with SBP <100 mm Hg and signs of shock.
- May cause tachyarrhythmias, fluctuations in blood pressure, headache, and nausea.
- Do not mix with sodium bicarbonate.

IV Administration

- Usual infusion rate is 2 to 20 mcg/kg per minute.
- Titrate so heart rate does not increase by >10% of baseline.
- Hemodynamic monitoring is recommended for optimal use.
- Elderly patients may have a significantly decreased response.

Advanced Cardiovascular Life Support Drugs

Drug/Therapy	Indications/Precautions	Adult Dosage
Dopamine IV infusion	**Indications** • Second-line drug for symptomatic bradycardia (after atropine). • Use for hypotension (SBP ≤70 to 100 mm Hg) with signs and symptoms of shock. **Precautions** • Correct hypovolemia with volume replacement before initiating dopamine. • Use with caution in cardiogenic shock with accompanying CHF. • May cause tachyarrhythmias, excessive vasoconstriction. • Do not mix with sodium bicarbonate.	**IV Administration** • Usual infusion rate is 2 to 20 mcg/kg per minute. • Titrate to patient response; taper slowly.

Epinephrine

Can be given via endotracheal tube

Available in 1:10 000 and 1:1000 concentrations

Indications

- **Cardiac arrest:** VF, pulseless VT, asystole, PEA.
- **Symptomatic bradycardia:** Can be considered after atropine as an alternative infusion to dopamine.
- **Severe hypotension:** Can be used when pacing and atropine fail, when hypotension accompanies bradycardia, or with phosphodiesterase enzyme inhibitor.
- **Anaphylaxis, severe allergic reactions:** Combine with large fluid volume, corticosteroids, antihistamines.

Precautions

- Raising blood pressure and increasing heart rate may cause myocardial ischemia, angina, and increased myocardial oxygen demand.
- High doses do not improve survival or neurologic outcome and may contribute to postresuscitation myocardial dysfunction.
- Higher doses *may* be required to treat poison/drug-induced shock.

Cardiac Arrest

- **IV/IO dose:** 1 mg (10 mL of 1:10 000 solution) administered every 3 to 5 minutes during resuscitation. Follow each dose with 20 mL flush, elevate arm for 10 to 20 seconds after dose.
- **Higher dose:** Higher doses (up to 0.2 mg/kg) may be used for specific indications (β-blocker or calcium channel blocker overdose).
- **Continuous infusion:** Initial rate: 0.1 to 0.5 mcg/kg per minute (for 70-kg patient: 7 to 35 mcg per minute); titrate to response.
- **Endotracheal route:** 2 to 2.5 mg diluted in 10 mL NS.

Profound Bradycardia or Hypotension
2 to 10 mcg per minute infusion; titrate to patient response.

Advanced Cardiovascular Life Support Drugs

Drug/Therapy	Indications/Precautions	Adult Dosage

Fibrinolytic Agents
 	
Alteplase, Recombinant (Activase); Tissue Plasminogen Activator (rtPA)
 	
50- and 100-mg vials reconstituted with sterile water to 1 mg/mL
 	
For all 4 agents, insert 2 peripheral IV lines; use 1 line exclusively for fibrinolytic administration
	Indications
	Cardiac arrest: Insufficient evidence to recommend routine use.
	
	AMI in adults (see ACS section):
	• ST elevation (>1 mm in ≥2 contiguous leads) or new or presumably new LBBB.
	• In context of signs and symptoms of AMI.
	• Time from onset of symptoms ≤12 hours.
	• See "Acute Coronary Syndromes: Fibrinolytic Checklist for STEMI" and Fibrinolytic Therapy under "ST-Segment Elevation Therapies: Fibrinolytic Strategy" for guidance on use of fibrinolytics in patients with STEMI.
	
	Acute ischemic stroke (see Stroke section):
	(Alteplase is the only fibrinolytic agent approved for acute ischemic stroke.)
	• Sudden onset of focal neurologic deficits or alterations in consciousness (eg, facial droop, arm drift, abnormal speech).
		Alteplase, Recombinant (rtPA)
		Recommended total dose is based on patient's weight.
		
		STEMI:
		• Accelerated infusion (1.5 hours)
		  — Give 15 mg IV bolus.
		  — Then 0.75 mg/kg over next 30 minutes (not to exceed 50 mg).
		  — Then 0.5 mg/kg over 60 minutes (not to exceed 35 mg).
		  — Maximum total dose: 100 mg.
		
		Acute ischemic stroke:
		• Give 0.9 mg/kg (maximum 90 mg) IV, infused over 60 minutes.
		• Give 10% of total dose as an initial IV bolus over 1 minute.
		• Give remaining 90% of total dose IV over next 60 minutes.

(continued)

Alteplase, Recombinant (Activase); Tissue Plasminogen Activator (rtPA)

- See "Use of IV rtPA for Acute Ischemic Stroke: Inclusion and Exclusion Characteristics" for guidance on which patients can be treated with rtPA based on time of symptom onset.

Reteplase, Recombinant (Retavase)
10-unit vials reconstituted with sterile water to 1 unit/mL

Streptokinase (Streptase)
Reconstitute to 1 mg/mL

Tenecteplase (TNKase)
50-mg vial reconstituted with sterile water

Precautions and Possible Exclusion Criteria for AMI in Adults/Acute Ischemic Stroke

- For AMI in adults, see "Acute Coronary Syndromes: Fibrinolytic Checklist for STEMI" and Fibrinolytic Therapy under "ST-Segment Elevation Therapies: Fibrinolytic Strategy" for indications, precautions, and contraindications.
- For acute ischemic stroke, see "Use of IV rtPA for Acute Ischemic Stroke: Inclusion and Exclusion Characteristics" for indications, precautions, and contraindications.

Reteplase, Recombinant
- Give first 10-unit IV bolus over 2 minutes.
- 30 minutes later give second 10-unit IV bolus over 2 minutes. (Give NS flush before and after each bolus.)

Streptokinase
1.5 million units in a 1-hour infusion.

Tenecteplase
- Bolus, weight adjusted
  - <60 kg: Give 30 mg.
  - 60-69 kg: Give 35 mg.
  - 70-79 kg: Give 40 mg.
  - 80-89 kg: Give 45 mg.
  - ≥90 kg: Give 50 mg.
- Administer single IV bolus over 5 seconds.
- Incompatible with dextrose solutions.

Advanced Cardiovascular Life Support Drugs

Drug/Therapy	Indications/Precautions	Adult Dosage
Flumazenil	**Indications** Reverse respiratory depression and sedative effects from pure benzodiazepine overdose. **Precautions** • Effects may not outlast effect of benzodiazepines. • Monitor for recurrent respiratory depression. • Do not use in suspected tricyclic overdose. • Do not use in seizure-prone patients, chronic benzodiazepine users, or alcoholics. • Do not use in unknown drug overdose or mixed drug overdose with drugs known to cause seizures (tricyclic antidepressants, cocaine, amphetamines, etc).	**First Dose** 0.2 mg IV over 15 seconds. **Second Dose** 0.3 mg IV over 30 seconds. If no adequate response, give third dose. **Third Dose** 0.5 mg IV given over 30 seconds. If no adequate response, repeat once every minute until adequate response or a total of 3 mg is given.

Furosemide

Powdered in 1-mg vials

Reconstitute with
provided solution

Indications
- For adjuvant therapy of acute pulmonary edema in patients with SBP >90 to 100 mm Hg (without signs and symptoms of shock).
- Hypertensive emergencies.

Precautions
Dehydration, hypovolemia, hypotension, hypokalemia, or other electrolyte imbalance may occur.

IV Administration
- 0.5 to 1 mg/kg given over 1 to 2 minutes.
- If no response, double dose to 2 mg/kg, given slowly over 1 to 2 minutes.
- For new-onset pulmonary edema with hypovolemia: <0.5 mg/kg.

Glucagon

Powdered in 1-mg vials

Reconstitute with
provided solution

Indications
Adjuvant treatment of toxic effects of calcium channel blocker or β-blocker.

Precautions
- May cause vomiting, hyperglycemia.

IV Infusion
3 to 10 mg IV slowly over 3 to 5 minutes, followed by infusion of 3 to 5 mg per hour.

Advanced Cardiovascular Life Support Drugs

Drug/Therapy	Indications/Precautions	Adult Dosage
Glycoprotein IIb/IIIa Inhibitors	**Indications** These drugs inhibit the integrin glycoprotein IIb/IIIa receptor in the membrane of platelets, inhibiting platelet aggregation. **Precautions/Contraindications** Active internal bleeding or bleeding disorder in past 30 days, history of intracranial hemorrhage or other bleeding, surgical procedure or trauma within 1 month, platelet count <150 000/mm³, hypersensitivity and concomitant use of another GP IIb/IIIa inhibitor (also see "ACS: Treatment for UA/NSTEMI").	*Note:* **Check package insert for current indications, doses, and duration of therapy.** Optimal duration of therapy has not been established.
Abciximab (ReoPro) *(continued)*	**Abciximab Indications** FDA approved for patients with NSTEMI or UA with planned PCI within 24 hours. **Abciximab Precautions/Contraindications** Must use with heparin. Binds irreversibly with platelets. Platelet function recovery requires 48 hours (regeneration). Readministration may cause hypersensitivity reaction.	**Abciximab** • **PCI:** 0.25 mg/kg IV bolus (10 to 60 minutes before procedure), then 0.125 mcg/kg per minute (to maximum of 10 mcg per minute) IV infusion for 12 hours.

Abciximab (ReoPro)
(continued)

- **ACS with planned PCI within 24 hours:**
0.25 mg/kg IV bolus, then
10 mcg per minute IV infusion for 18 to
24 hours, concluding 1 hour after PCI.

Eptifibatide (Integrilin)

Eptifibatide Indications

For high-risk UA/NSTEMI and patients
undergoing PCI.

Actions/Precautions

Platelet function recovers within 4 to 8 hours
after discontinuation.

Eptifibatide

- **PCI:** 180 mcg/kg IV bolus over
1 to 2 minutes, then begin 2 mcg/kg
per minute IV infusion, then repeat
bolus in 10 minutes.
- Maximum dose (121-kg patient) for PCI:
22.6 mg bolus; 15 mg per hour infusion.
- Infusion duration 18 to 24 hours
after PCI.
- Reduce rate of infusion by 50% if
creatinine clearance <50 mL per minute.

Tirofiban (Aggrastat)

Tirofiban Indications

For high-risk UA/NSTEMI and patients
undergoing PCI.

Actions/Precautions

Platelet function recovers within 4 to 8 hours
after discontinuation.

Tirofiban

- **PCI:** 0.4 mcg/kg per minute IV for 30
minutes, then 0.1 mcg/kg per minute IV
infusion (for 18 to 24 hours after PCI).
- Reduce rate of infusion by 50% if
creatinine clearance <30 mL per minute.

Advanced Cardiovascular Life Support Drugs

Drug/Therapy	Indications/Precautions	Adult Dosage
Fondaparinux (Arixtra)	**Indications** • For use in ACS. • To inhibit thrombin generation by factor Xa inhibition. • May be used for anticoagulation in patients with history of heparin-induced thrombocytopenia. **Precautions/Contraindications** • Hemorrhage may complicate therapy. • Contraindicated in patients with creatinine clearance <30 mL per minute; use with caution in patients with creatinine clearance 30 to 50 mL per minute. • Increased risk of catheter thrombosis in patients undergoing PCI; coadministration of unfractionated heparin required.	**STEMI Protocol** • Initial dose 2.5 mg IV bolus followed by 2.5 mg subcutaneously every 24 hours for up to 8 days. **UA/NSTEMI Protocol** • 2.5 mg subcutaneously every 24 hours.

Heparin, Unfractionated (UFH)

Concentrations range from 1000 to 40 000 units/mL

Indications
- Adjuvant therapy in AMI.
- Begin heparin with fibrin-specific lytics (eg, alteplase, reteplase, tenecteplase).

Precautions/Contraindications
- Same contraindications as for fibrinolytic therapy: active bleeding; recent intracranial, intraspinal, or eye surgery; severe hypertension; bleeding disorders; gastrointestinal bleeding.
- Doses and laboratory targets appropriate when used with fibrinolytic therapy.
- Do not use if platelet count is or falls below <100 000 or with history of heparin-induced thrombocytopenia. For these patients consider direct antithrombins. See bivalirudin on the next page.

UFH IV Infusion—STEMI
- Initial bolus 60 units/kg (maximum bolus: 4000 units).
- Continue 12 units/kg per hour, round to the nearest 50 units (maximum initial rate: 1000 units per hour).
- Adjust to maintain aPTT 1.5 to 2 times the control values (50 to 70 seconds) for 48 hours or until angiography.
- Check initial aPTT at 3 hours, then every 6 hours until stable, then daily.
- Follow institutional heparin protocol.
- Platelet count daily.

UFH IV Infusion—UA/NSTEMI
- Initial bolus 60 units/kg. Maximum: 4000 units.
- 12 units/kg per hour. Maximum initial rate: 1000 units per hour.
- Follow institutional protocol (see Heparin in ACS section).

49

Advanced Cardiovascular Life Support Drugs

Drug/Therapy	Indications/Precautions	Adult Dosage
Heparin, Low Molecular Weight (LMWH)	**Indications** For use in ACS, specifically patients with UA/NSTEMI. These drugs inhibit thrombin generation by factor Xa inhibition and also inhibit thrombin indirectly by formation of a complex with antithrombin III. These drugs are **not** neutralized by heparin-binding proteins. **Precautions** • Hemorrhage may complicate any therapy with LMWH. Contraindicated in presence of hypersensitivity to heparin or pork products or history of sensitivity to drug. Use **enoxaparin** with extreme caution in patients with type II heparin-induced thrombocytopenia. • Adjust dose for renal insufficiency. • Contraindicated if platelet count <100 000. For these patients consider direct antithrombins. **Heparin Reversal** ICH or life-threatening bleed: Administer protamine; refer to package insert.	**STEMI Protocol** • Enoxaparin — Age <75 years, normal creatinine clearance: initial bolus 30 mg IV with second bolus 15 minutes later of 1 mg/kg subcutaneously, repeat every 12 hours (maximum 100 mg/dose for first 2 doses). — Age ≥75 years: Eliminate initial IV bolus, give 0.75 mg/kg subcutaneously every 12 hours (maximum 75 mg/dose for first 2 doses). — If creatinine clearance <30 mL per minute, give 1 mg/kg subcutaneously every 24 hours. **UA/NSTEMI Protocol** • Enoxaparin: Loading dose 30 mg IV bolus. Maintenance dose 1 mg/kg subcutaneously every 12 hours. If creatinine clearance <30 mL per minute, give every 24 hours. • Bivalirudin: Bolus with 0.1 mg/kg IV; then begin infusion of 0.25 mg/kg per hour.

Ibutilide

Intervention of choice is
DC cardioversion

Indications

Treatment of supraventricular arrhythmias,
including atrial fibrillation and atrial flutter
when duration ≤48 hours. Short duration of
action. Effective for the conversion of atrial
fibrillation or flutter of relatively brief duration.

Precautions/Contraindications

Contraindication: Do not give to patients
with QT$_c$ >440 milliseconds. Ventricular
arrhythmias develop in approximately
2% to 5% of patients (polymorphic VT,
including torsades de pointes). *Monitor
ECG continuously for arrhythmias during
administration and for 4 to 6 hours after
administration with defibrillator nearby.*
Patients with significantly impaired LV
function are at highest risk for arrhythmias.

Dose for Adults ≥60 kg

1 mg (10 mL) administered IV (diluted
or undiluted) over 10 minutes. A second
dose may be administered at the same
rate 10 minutes later.

Dose for Adults <60 kg

0.01 mg/kg initial IV dose administered
over 10 minutes.

Advanced Cardiovascular Life Support Drugs

Drug/Therapy	Indications/Precautions	Adult Dosage
Inamrinone Phosphodiesterase enzyme inhibitor	**Indications** Severe congestive heart failure refractory to diuretics, vasodilators, and conventional inotropic agents. **Precautions** • Do not mix with dextrose solutions or other drugs. • May cause tachyarrhythmias, hypotension, or thrombocytopenia. • Can increase myocardial ischemia.	**IV Loading Dose and Infusion** • 0.75 mg/kg (not to exceed 1 mg/kg) given over 2 to 3 minutes. Give loading dose over 10 to 15 minutes with LV dysfunction (eg, postresuscitation). • Follow with infusion of 5 to 15 mcg/kg per minute titrated to clinical effect. • Additional bolus may be given in 30 minutes. • Requires hemodynamic monitoring. • Creatinine clearance <10 mL per minute: reduce dose 25% to 50%.

Isoproterenol

IV infusion

Indications

- *Use cautiously as temporizing measure if external pacer is not available* for treatment of symptomatic bradycardia.
- Refractory torsades de pointes unresponsive to magnesium sulfate.
- *Temporary* control of bradycardia in heart transplant patients (denervated heart unresponsive to atropine).
- Poisoning from β-blockers.

Precautions

- Do not use for treatment of cardiac arrest.
- Increases myocardial oxygen requirements, which may increase myocardial ischemia.
- Do not give with epinephrine; can cause VF/VT.
- Do not give to patients with poison/drug-induced shock (except for β-blocker poisoning).
- May use higher doses for β-blocker poisoning.

IV Administration

- Infuse at 2 to 10 mcg per minute.
- Titrate to adequate heart rate.
- In torsades de pointes titrate to increase heart rate until VT is suppressed.

51

Drug/Therapy	Indications/Precautions	Adult Dosage
Lidocaine Can be given via endotracheal tube	**Indications** • Alternative to amiodarone in cardiac arrest from VF/VT. • Stable monomorphic VT with preserved ventricular function. • Stable polymorphic VT with normal baseline QT interval and preserved LV function when ischemia is treated and electrolyte balance is corrected. • Can be used for stable polymorphic VT with baseline QT-interval prolongation if torsades suspected. **Precautions/Contraindications** • **Contraindication:** *Prophylactic* use in AMI is contraindicated. • Reduce maintenance dose (not loading dose) in presence of impaired liver function or LV dysfunction. • Discontinue infusion immediately if signs of toxicity develop.	**Cardiac Arrest From VF/VT** • Initial dose: 1 to 1.5 mg/kg IV/IO. • For refractory VF may give additional 0.5 to 0.75 mg/kg IV push, repeat in 5 to 10 minutes; maximum 3 doses or total of 3 mg/kg. **Perfusing Arrhythmia** For stable VT, wide-complex tachycardia of uncertain type, significant ectopy: • Doses ranging from 0.5 to 0.75 mg/kg and up to 1 to 1.5 mg/kg may be used. • Repeat 0.5 to 0.75 mg/kg every 5 to 10 minutes; maximum total dose: 3 mg/kg. **Maintenance Infusion** 1 to 4 mg per minute (30 to 50 mcg/kg per minute).

Magnesium Sulfate

Indications

- Recommended for use in cardiac arrest only if torsades de pointes or suspected hypomagnesemia is present.
- Life-threatening ventricular arrhythmias due to digitalis toxicity.
- Routine administration in hospitalized patients with AMI is **not** recommended.

Precautions

- Occasional fall in blood pressure with rapid administration.
- Use with caution if renal failure is present.

Cardiac Arrest (Due to Hypomagnesemia or Torsades de Pointes)

1 to 2 g (2 to 4 mL of a 50% solution) diluted in 10 mL of D_5W IV/IO.

Torsades de Pointes With a Pulse or AMI With Hypomagnesemia

- Loading dose of 1 to 2 g mixed in 50 to 100 mL of D_5W, over 5 to 60 minutes IV.
- Follow with 0.5 to 1 g per hour IV (titrate to control torsades).

Mannitol

Strengths: 5%, 10%, 15%, 20%, and 25%

Indications

Increased intracranial pressure in management of neurologic emergencies.

Precautions

- Monitor fluid status and serum osmolality (not to exceed 310 mOsm/kg).
- Caution in renal failure because fluid overload may result.

IV Administration

- Administer 0.5 to 1 g/kg over 5 to 10 minutes through in-line filter.
- Additional doses of 0.25 to 2 g/kg can be given every 4 to 6 hours as needed.
- Use with support of oxygenation and ventilation.

Advanced Cardiovascular Life Support Drugs

Drug/Therapy	Indications/Precautions	Adult Dosage
Milrinone Shorter half-life than inamrinone	**Indications** Myocardial dysfunction and increased systemic or pulmonary vascular resistance, including • Congestive heart failure in postoperative cardiovascular surgical patients. • Shock with high systemic vascular resistance. **Precautions** May produce nausea, vomiting, hypotension, particularly in volume-depleted patients. Shorter half-life and less effect on platelets but more risk for ventricular arrhythmia than inamrinone. Drug may accumulate in renal failure and in patients with low cardiac output; reduce dose in renal failure.	**Loading Dose** 50 mcg/kg over 10 minutes IV loading dose. **IV Infusion** • 0.375 to 0.75 mcg/kg per minute. • Hemodynamic monitoring required. • Reduce dose in renal impairment.
Morphine Sulfate *(continued)*	**Indications** • Chest pain with ACS unresponsive to nitrates. • Acute cardiogenic pulmonary edema (if blood pressure is adequate).	**IV Administration** • STEMI: Give 2 to 4 mg IV. May give additional doses of 2 to 8 mg IV at 5- to 15-minute intervals. Analgesic of choice.

Morphine Sulfate
(continued)

Precautions
- Administer slowly and titrate to effect.
- May cause respiratory depression.
- Causes hypotension in volume-depleted patients.
- Use with caution in RV infarction.
- May reverse with naloxone (0.04 to 2 mg IV).

- UA/NSTEMI: Give 1 to 5 mg IV only if symptoms not relieved by nitrates or if symptoms recur. Use with caution.

Naloxone Hydrochloride

Can be given via entotracheal tube

Indications
Respiratory and neurologic depression due to opiate intoxication unresponsive to oxygen and support of ventilation.

Precautions
- May cause severe opiate withdrawal, including hypertensive crisis and pulmonary edema when given in large doses (titration of small doses recommended).
- Half-life shorter than narcotics, repeat dosing may be needed.
- Monitor for recurrent respiratory depression.
- Rare anaphylactic reactions have been reported.
- Assist ventilation before naloxone administration, avoid sympathetic stimulation.
- Avoid in meperidine-induced seizures.

Administration
- Typical IV dose 0.04 to 0.4 mg, titrate until ventilation adequate.
- Use higher doses for complete narcotic reversal.
- Can administer up to 6 to 10 mg over short period (<10 minutes).
- If total reversal is not required (eg, respiratory depression from sedation), smaller doses of 0.04 mg repeated every 2 to 3 minutes may be used.
- IM/subcutaneously: 0.4 to 0.8 mg.
- For chronic opioid-addicted patients, use smaller dose and titrate slowly.

Advanced Cardiovascular Life Support Drugs

Drug/Therapy	Indications/Precautions	Adult Dosage
Nicardipine (Cardene) Calcium channel blocker	**Indications** • Hypertensive emergencies. • Decrease blood pressure to ≤185/110 mm Hg before administration of fibrinolytic therapy. **Precautions/Contraindications** • Avoid rapid decrease in blood pressure. • Reflex tachycardia or increased angina may occur in patients with extensive coronary disease. • Avoid use in patients with severe aortic stenosis. • Do not mix with sodium bicarbonate or Ringer's lactate solution.	**Acute Hypertension Emergencies** • Initial infusion rate 5 mg per hour; may increase by 2.5 mg per hour every 5 to 15 minutes to maximum of 15 mg per hour. • Decrease infusion rate to 3 mg per hour once desired blood pressure reached. →
Nitroglycerin Available in IV form, sublingual tablets, and aerosol spray *(continued)*	**Indications** • Initial antianginal for suspected ischemic pain. • For initial 24 to 48 hours in patients with *AMI and CHF*, large anterior wall infarction, persistent or recurrent ischemia, or hypertension. →	**IV Administration** • **IV bolus:** 12.5 to 25 mcg (if no SL or spray given).

Nitroglycerin
(continued)

- Continued use (beyond 48 hours) for patients with recurrent angina or persistent pulmonary congestion (nitrate-free interval recommended).
- Hypertensive urgency with ACS.

Contraindications

- Hypotension (SBP <90 mm Hg or ≥30 mm Hg below baseline).
- Severe bradycardia (<50 per minute) or tachycardia (>100 per minute).
- RV infarction.
- Use of phosphodiesterase inhibitors for erectile dysfunction (eg, sildenafil and vardenafil within 24 hours; tadalafil within 48 hours).

Precautions

- Generally, with evidence of AMI and normotension, do not reduce SBP to <110 mm Hg. If patient is hypertensive, do not decrease mean arterial pressure (MAP) by >25% (from initial MAP).
- Do not mix with other drugs.
- Patient should sit or lie down when receiving this medication.
- Do not shake aerosol spray because this affects metered dose.

- **Infusion:** Begin at 10 mcg per minute. Titrate to effect, increase by 10 mcg per minute every 3 to 5 minutes until desired effect. Ceiling dose of 200 mcg per minute commonly used.
  — Route of choice for emergencies.

Sublingual Route

- 1 tablet (0.3 to 0.4 mg), repeated for total of 3 doses at 5-minute intervals.
- 1 to 2 sprays for 0.5 to 1 second at 5-minute intervals (provides 0.4 mg per dose). Maximum 3 sprays within 15 minutes.
- *Note:* Patients should be instructed to contact EMS if pain is unrelieved or increasing after 1 tablet or sublingual spray.

Advanced Cardiovascular Life Support Drugs

Drug/Therapy	Indications/Precautions	Adult Dosage
Nitroprusside (Sodium Nitroprusside)	**Indications** • Hypertensive crisis. • To reduce afterload in heart failure and acute pulmonary edema. • To reduce afterload in acute mitral or aortic valve regurgitation. **Precautions** • May cause hypotension and cyanide toxicity. • May reverse hypoxic pulmonary vasoconstriction in patients with pulmonary disease, exacerbating intrapulmonary shunting, resulting in hypoxemia. • Other side effects include headaches, nausea, vomiting, and abdominal cramps. • Contraindicated in patients who have recently taken phosphodiesterase inhibitors for erectile dysfunction (eg, sildenafil).	**IV Administration** • Add 50 or 100 mg to 250 mL D₅W. (Refer to your institutional pharmacy policy.) • Begin at 0.1 mcg/kg per minute and titrate upward every 3 to 5 minutes to desired effect (usually up to 5 mcg/kg per minute, but higher doses up to 10 mcg/kg may be needed). • Use with an infusion pump; use hemodynamic monitoring for optimal safety. • Action occurs within 1 to 2 minutes. • Light sensitive; cover drug reservoir and tubing with opaque material.

Norepinephrine

Indications

- Severe cardiogenic shock and hemodynamically significant hypotension (SBP <70 mm Hg) with low total peripheral resistance.
- Agent of last resort for management of ischemic heart disease and shock.

Precautions

- Increases myocardial oxygen requirements; raises blood pressure and heart rate.
- May induce arrhythmias. Use with caution in patients with acute ischemia; monitor cardiac output.
- Extravasation causes tissue necrosis.
- If extravasation occurs, administer phentolamine 5 to 10 mg in 10 to 15 mL saline solution; infiltrate into area.
- Relatively contraindicated in patients with hypovolemia.

IV Administration (Only Route)

- Initial rate: 0.1 to 0.5 mcg/kg per minute (for 70-kg patient: 7 to 35 mcg per minute); titrate to response.
- Do not administer in same IV line as alkaline solutions.
- Poison/drug-induced hypotension may require higher doses to achieve adequate perfusion.

Advanced Cardiovascular Life Support Drugs

Oxygen

Drug/Therapy

Delivered from portable tanks or installed, wall-mounted sources through delivery devices

Indications/Precautions

Indications

- Any suspected cardiopulmonary emergency.
- Complaints of shortness of breath and suspected ischemic pain.
- For ACS: May administer to all patients until stable. Continue if pulmonary congestion, ongoing ischemia, or oxygen saturation <94%.
- For patients with suspected stroke and hypoxemia, arterial oxygen desaturation (oxyhemoglobin saturation <94%), or unknown oxyhemoglobin saturation. May consider administration to patients who are not hypoxemic.
- After ROSC following resuscitation: Use the minimum inspired oxygen concentration to achieve oxyhemoglobin saturation ≥94%. If equipment available, wean inspired oxygen to avoid hyperoxia, when inspired oxygen when oxyhemoglobin saturation is 100% but maintain ≥94%.

Adult Dosage

Device	Flow Rate	O₂ (%)
Nasal cannula	1-6 L per minute	21-44
Venturi mask	4-12 L per minute	24-50
Partial rebreathing mask	6-10 L per minute	35-60
Nonrebreathing oxygen mask with reservoir	6-15 L per minute	60-100
Bag-mask with nonrebreathing "tail"	15 L per minute	95-100

(continued)

Oxygen
(continued)

Precautions

- Observe closely when using with pulmonary patients known to be dependent on hypoxic respiratory drive (very rare).
- Pulse oximetry may be inaccurate in low cardiac output states, with vasoconstriction, or with exposure to carbon monoxide.

Note: Pulse oximetry provides a useful method of titrating oxygen administration to maintain physiologic oxygen saturation (see Precautions).

Advanced Cardiovascular Life Support Drugs

Drug/Therapy	Indications/Precautions	Adult Dosage

Procainamide	**Indications**
	• Useful for treatment of a wide variety of arrhythmias, including stable monomorphic VT with normal QT interval and preserved LV function.
	• May use for treatment of reentry SVT uncontrolled by adenosine and vagal maneuvers if blood pressure stable.
	• Stable wide-complex tachycardia of unknown origin.
	• Atrial fibrillation with rapid rate in Wolff-Parkinson-White syndrome.
	
	Precautions
	• If cardiac or renal dysfunction is present, reduce maximum total dose to 12 mg/kg and maintenance infusion to 1 to 2 mg per minute.
	• Proarrhythmic, especially in setting of AMI, hypokalemia, or hypomagnesemia.
	• May induce hypotension in patients with impaired LV function.
	• Use with caution with other drugs that prolong QT interval (eg, amiodarone). Expert consultation advised.
		Recurrent VF/VT
		• 20 mg per minute IV infusion (maximum total dose: 17 mg/kg).
		• In urgent situations, up to 50 mg per minute may be administered to total dose of 17 mg/kg.
		
		Other Indications
		• 20 mg per minute IV infusion until one of the following occurs:
		  — Arrhythmia suppression.
		  — Hypotension.
		  — QRS widens by >50%.
		  — Total dose of 17 mg/kg is given.
		• Use in cardiac arrest limited by need for slow infusion and uncertain efficacy.
		
		Maintenance Infusion
		1 to 4 mg per minute (dilute in D_5W or NS). Reduce dose in presence of renal insufficiency.

Sodium Bicarbonate

Indications

- Known preexisting hyperkalemia.
- Known preexisting bicarbonate-responsive acidosis; eg, diabetic ketoacidosis or overdose of tricyclic antidepressant, aspirin, cocaine, or diphenhydramine.
- Prolonged resuscitation with effective ventilation; on return of spontaneous circulation after long arrest interval.
- Not useful or effective in hypercarbic acidosis (eg, cardiac arrest and CPR without intubation).

Precautions

- Adequate ventilation and CPR, not bicarbonate, are the major "buffer agents" in cardiac arrest.
- Not recommended for routine use in cardiac arrest patients.

IV Administration

- 1 mEq/kg IV bolus.
- If rapidly available, use arterial blood gas analysis to guide bicarbonate therapy (calculated base deficits or bicarbonate concentration). During cardiac arrest, ABG results are not reliable indicators of acidosis.

Drug/Therapy	Indications/Precautions	Adult Dosage
Sotalol Seek expert consultation	**Indications** Treatment of supraventricular arrhythmias and ventricular arrhythmias in patients without structural heart disease. **Precautions/Contraindications** • Should be avoided in patients with poor perfusion because of significant negative inotropic effects. • Adverse effects include bradycardia, hypotension, and arrhythmias (torsades de pointes). • Use with caution with other drugs that prolong QT interval (eg, procainamide, amiodarone). • May become toxic in patients with renal impairment; contraindicated if creatinine clearance <40 mL per minute.	**IV Administration** • 1 to 1.5 mg/kg. • Check hospital protocol for infusion rate. Package insert recommends slow infusion, but literature supports more rapid infusion of 1.5 mg/kg over 5 minutes or less.
Thienopyridines (see *ADP Antagonists*)		
Thrombolytic Agents (see *Fibrinolytic Agents*)		

Vasopressin

Can be given via endotracheal tube

Indications

- May be used as alternative pressor to epinephrine in treatment of adult shock-refractory VF.
- May be useful alternative to epinephrine in asystole, PEA.
- May be useful for hemodynamic support in vasodilatory shock (eg, septic shock).

Precautions/Contraindications

- Potent peripheral vasoconstrictor. Increased peripheral vascular resistance may provoke cardiac ischemia and angina.
- Not recommended for responsive patients with coronary artery disease.

IV Administration

Cardiac arrest: One dose of 40 units IV/IO push may replace either first or second dose of epinephrine. Epinephrine can be administered every 3 to 5 minutes during cardiac arrest.

Vasodilatory shock: Continuous infusion of 0.02 to 0.04 units per minute.

Advanced Cardiovascular Life Support Drugs

Drug/Therapy	Indications/Precautions	Adult Dosage
Verapamil	**Indications** • Alternative drug (after adenosine) to terminate re-entry SVT with narrow QRS complex and adequate blood pressure and *preserved LV function.* • May control ventricular response in patients with atrial fibrillation, flutter, or multifocal atrial tachycardia. **Precautions** • Give *only* to patients with narrow-complex reentry SVT or known supraventricular arrhythmias. • Do not use for wide-QRS tachycardias of uncertain origin, and avoid use for Wolff-Parkinson-White syndrome and atrial fibrillation, sick sinus syndrome, or second- or third-degree AV block without pacemaker. • May decrease myocardial contractility and can produce peripheral vasodilation and hypotension. IV calcium may restore blood pressure in toxic cases. • Concurrent IV administration with IV β-blockers may produce severe hypotension. Use with extreme caution in patients receiving oral β-blockers.	**IV Administration** • **First dose:** 2.5 to 5 mg IV bolus over 2 minutes (over 3 minutes in older patients). • **Second dose:** 5 to 10 mg, if needed, every 15 to 30 minutes. Maximum total dose: 20 mg. • **Alternative:** 5 mg bolus every 15 minutes to total dose of 30 mg.

Useful Calculations and Formulas

Calculation	Formula	Comments
Anion gap (serum concentration in mEq/L)	$[Na^+] - ([Cl^-] + [HCO_3^-])$	Normal range: 10 to 15 mEq/L. A gap >15 suggests metabolic acidosis.
Osmolal gap	$Osmolality_{measured} - Osmolality_{calculated}$ Normal = <10	Osmolal gap normally <10. If osmolal gap is >10, suspect unknown osmotically active substances.
Calculated osmolality (in mOsm/L)	$(2 \times [Na^+]) + ([Glucose] \div 18) + ([BUN] \div 2.8)$	Simplified to give *effective* osmolality. Normal = 272 to 300 mOsm/L
Total free water deficit (in L)	$\dfrac{([Na^+]_{measured} - 140)}{140} \times TBW$ $TBW_{in\,L} = (0.6_{men}\ or\ 0.5_{women}) \times Weight_{in\,kg}$	Use to calculate quantity of water needed to correct water deficit in hypernatremia.

Sodium deficit (in total mEq)	$([Na^+]_{desired} - [Na^+]_{measured}) \times TBW_{in\,L}$ $TBW_{in\,L} = (0.6_{men}\ \text{or}\ 0.5_{women}) \times Weight_{in\,kg}$	Use to calculate sodium deficit that is partially treated with 3% saline in severe hyponatremia (3% saline contains 513 mEq sodium per liter). Plan to raise serum sodium: • Asymptomatic: 0.5 mEq/L per hour • Neurologic symptoms: 1 mEq/L per hour until symptoms are controlled • Seizures: 2 to 4 mEq/L per hour until seizures are controlled
Determination of *predicted* pH	$(40 - PCO_2) \times 0.008 = \pm\Delta$ in pH from 7.4	For every 1 mm Hg uncompensated change in PCO_2 from 40, pH will change by 0.008. Measured pH less than predicted pH: metabolic acidosis is present. Measured pH greater than predicted pH: metabolic alkalosis is present.

Emergency Treatments and Treatment Sequence for Hyperkalemia

Therapy	Dose	Effect Mechanism	Onset of Effect	Duration of Effect
Calcium	• Calcium chloride (10%): 5 to 10 mL IV • Calcium gluconate (10%): 15 to 30 mL IV	• Antagonism of toxic effects of hyperkalemia at cell membrane	• 1 to 3 min	• 30 to 60 min
Sodium bicarbonate	• Begin with 50 mEq IV • May repeat in 15 minutes	• Redistribution: intracellular shift	• 5 to 10 min	• 1 to 2 h
Insulin plus glucose (use 2 units insulin per 5 g glucose)	• 10 units regular insulin IV plus 25 g dextrose (50 mL D_{50})	• Redistribution: intracellular shift	• 30 min	• 4 to 6 h

Nebulized albuterol	• 10 to 20 mg over 15 min • May repeat	• Redistribution: intracellular shift	• 15 min	• 15 to 90 min
Diuresis with furosemide	• 40 to 80 mg IV bolus	• Removal from body	• At start of diuresis	• Until end of diuresis
Cation-exchange resin (Kayexalate)	• 15 to 50 g PO or PR plus sorbitol	• Removal from body	• 1 to 2 h	• 4 to 6 h
Peritoneal or hemodialysis	• Per institutional protocol	• Removal from body	• At start of dialysis	• Until end of dialysis

Common Toxidromes*

Whenever possible, contact a medical toxicologist or poison center (eg, in USA: 1-800-222-1222) for advice when treating suspected severe poisoning.

Cardiac Signs

Tachycardia and/or Hypertension	Bradycardia and/or Hypotension	Cardiac Conduction Delays (Wide QRS)
• Amphetamines • Anticholinergic drugs • Antihistamines • Cocaine • Theophylline/caffeine • Withdrawal states	• β-Blockers • Calcium channel blockers • Clonidine • Digoxin and related glycosides • Organophosphates and carbamates	• Cocaine • Cyclic antidepressants • Local anesthetics • Propoxyphene • Vaughan-Williams Class Ia and Ic agents (eg, quinidine, flecainide)

CNS/Metabolic Signs

Seizures	CNS and/or Respiratory Depression	Metabolic Acidosis
• Cyclic antidepressants • Isoniazid • Selective and nonselective norepinephrine reuptake inhibitors (eg, bupropion) • Withdrawal states	• Antidepressants (several classes) • Benzodiazepines • Carbon monoxide • Ethanol • Methanol • Opioids • Oral hypoglycemics	• Cyanide • Ethylene glycol • Iron • Metformin • Methanol • Salicylates

*Differential diagnosis lists are partial.

Rapid Dosing Guide for Antidotes Used in Emergency Cardiovascular Care for Treatment of Toxic Ingestions

Whenever possible, consult a medical toxicologist or call poison center (eg, in USA: 1-800-222-1222) for advice before administering antidotes.

Antidote	Common Indications: Toxicity due to	Adult Dose*	Pediatric Dose* Do not exceed adult dose.	Notes
Atropine	• β-Blockers • Calcium channel blockers • Clonidine • Digoxin	0.5-1 mg IV every 2-3 minutes	0.02 mg/kg IV (minimum dose 0.1 mg) every 2-3 minutes	Use for hemodynamically significant bradycardia. Higher doses often required for organo-phosphate or carbamate poisoning.
Calcium	• β-Blockers • Calcium channel blockers	• Calcium chloride (10%): 1-2 g (10-20 mL) IV • Calcium gluconate (10%): 3-6 g (30-60 mL) IV • Follow initial dose with same dose by continuous hourly infusion	• Calcium chloride (10%): 20 mg/kg (0.2 mL/kg) IV • Calcium gluconate (10%): 60 mg/kg (0.6 mL/kg) IV • Follow initial dose with same dose by continuous hourly infusion	Use for hypotension. Avoid calcium chloride when possible if using peripheral IV, particularly in children. Higher doses may be required for calcium channel blocker overdose (use caution and monitor serum calcium).

*These doses are often different from doses used in other emergency cardiovascular care situations. The ideal dose has not been determined for many indications; the doses above may not be ideal. Most antidotes may be repeated as needed to achieve and maintain the desired clinical effect. Unless otherwise noted, IV doses may also be given via the IO route. Contact medical toxicologist, call poison center (eg, in USA: 1-800-222-1222), or refer to written treatment guidance for specific dosing advice.

(continued)

Rapid Dosing Guide for Antidotes Used in Emergency Cardiovascular Care for Treatment of Toxic Ingestions (continued)

Antidote	Common Indications: Toxicity due to	Adult Dose*	Pediatric Dose* Do not exceed adult dose.	Notes
Digoxin Immune Fab	• Digoxin and related glycosides	• **If amount of digoxin ingested is known:** Give 1 vial IV for every 0.5 mg digoxin ingested. • **If amount of digoxin ingested is unknown or if chronic intoxication with a known digoxin level:** Dose (vials, administered IV) = $$\frac{\text{(serum digoxin concentration [ng/mL]} \times \text{weight [kg])}}{100}$$ • **Unknown dose and level, cardiovascular collapse:** 10-20 vials IV		
Flumazenil	• Benzodiazepines	0.2 mg IV every 15 seconds, up to 3 mg total dose	0.01 mg/kg IV every 15 seconds, up to 0.05 mg/kg total dose	Do not use for unknown overdose, suspected TCA overdose, or patients who are benzodiazepine dependent due to risk of precipitating seizures.
Glucagon	• β-Blockers • Calcium channel blockers	3-10 mg IV bolus, followed by 3-5 mg per hour IV infusion	0.05-0.15 mg/kg IV bolus, followed by 0.05-0.10 mg/kg per hour IV infusion	Bolus often causes vomiting.

Hydroxo-cobalamin	• Cyanide	5 g IV	Dilute in 100 mL normal saline; infuse over 15 minutes. Toxicologist or other specialist may follow with sodium thiosulfate (separate IV).
Lipid Emulsion	• Local anesthetics • Calcium channel blockers • β-Blockers • Other drugs	1.5 mL/kg of 20% long-chain fatty acid solution IV bolus, followed by 0.25 mL/kg per minute IV infusion for 30-60 minutes	70 mg/kg IV
Insulin	• β-Blockers • Calcium channel blockers	1 unit/kg IV bolus, then 0.5-1 units/kg per hour IV infusion, titrated to blood pressure	Give dextrose 0.5 g/kg with insulin. Start dextrose infusion 0.5 g/kg per hour and check blood sugar frequently. Replace potassium to maintain serum potassium 2.5-2.8 mEq/L.

*These doses are often different from doses used in other emergency cardiovascular care situations. The ideal dose has not been determined for many indications; the doses above may not be ideal. Most antidotes may be repeated as needed to achieve and maintain the desired clinical effect. Unless otherwise noted, IV doses may also be given via the IO route. Contact medical toxicologist, call poison center (eg, in USA: 1-800-222-1222), or refer to written treatment guidance for specific dosing advice.

(continued)

Rapid Dosing Guide for Antidotes Used in Emergency Cardiovascular Care for Treatment of Toxic Ingestions (continued)

Antidote	Common Indications: Toxicity due to	Adult Dose*	Pediatric Dose* Do not exceed adult dose.	Notes
Naloxone	• Opioids	0.04-0.4 mg IV; repeat every 2-3 minutes and escalate dose as needed to maximum 10 mg	0.1 mg/kg IV (up to 2 mg per dose). Repeat every 2-3 minutes. For partial reversal of respiratory depression (eg, procedural sedation), 0.001-0.005 mg/kg (1-5 mcg/kg) IV. Titrate to effect.	Use only for respiratory depression or loss of airway reflexes. May also be given by IM, IO, intranasal, or endotracheal routes.
Sodium Bicarbonate	• Cyclic antidepressants	1 mEq/kg IV (1 mL/kg of 8.4% solution); consider infusion following initial dose		Repeat as needed until QRS narrows. Avoid sodium >155 mEq/L or pH >7.55. Dilute before administration in small children.

Sodium Nitrite	• Cyanide	300 mg IV over 3-5 minutes (10 mL of 3% solution)	10 mg/kg (0.33 mL/kg of 10% solution) IV over 3-5 minutes	Hydroxocobalamin preferred to sodium nitrite, if available. May give inhaled amyl nitrite as temporizing measure while establishing vascular access. Follow with sodium thiosulfate administration. Reduced dose required for children with anemia.
Sodium Thiosulfate	• Cyanide	12.5 g (50 mL of 25% solution) IV over 10 minutes	400 mg/kg (1.65 mL/kg of 25% solution) IV over 10 minutes	Use separate IV from hydroxocobalamin. Consider expert consultation.

*These doses are often different from doses used in other emergency cardiovascular care situations. The ideal dose has not been determined for many indications; the doses above may not be ideal. Most antidotes may be repeated as needed to achieve and maintain the desired clinical effect. Unless otherwise noted, IV doses may also be given via the IO route. Contact medical toxicologist, call poison center (eg, in USA: 1-800-222-1222), or refer to written treatment guidance for specific dosing advice.

Rapid Sequence Intubation

Pre-event Equipment Checklist for Endotracheal Intubation

☐	Universal precautions (gloves, mask, eye protection)
☐	Cardiac monitor, pulse oximeter, and blood pressure monitoring device
☐	Continuous waveform capnography device or, if not available, exhaled CO_2 detector (qualitative) or esophageal detector device (aspiration technique)
☐	Intravenous and intraosseous infusion equipment
☐	Oxygen supply, bag mask (appropriate size)
☐	Oral/tracheal suction equipment (appropriate size); confirm that it is working
☐	Oral and nasopharyngeal airways (appropriate size)
☐	Endotracheal tubes with stylets (all sizes) and sizes 0.5 mm (i.d.) above and below anticipated size for patient
☐	Laryngoscope (curved and straight blades) and/or video laryngoscope; backup laryngoscope available
☐	10-mL syringes to test inflate endotracheal tube balloon
☐	Adhesive/cloth tape or commercial endotracheal tube holder to secure tube
☐	Towels, sheets, or pad to align airway by placing under head or torso
☐	Rescue equipment as needed for difficult airway management or anticipated complications (eg, supraglottic airway, transtracheal ventilation, and/or cricothyrotomy equipment)

RSI Protocol

Pre-event preparation	1. Obtain brief medical history and perform focused physical examination. 2. Prepare equipment, monitors, personnel, medications. 3. If neck injury not suspected: place in sniffing position. If neck injury suspected: stabilize cervical spine.
Preoxygenate	4. Preoxygenate with FiO_2 of 100% by mask (nonrebreather preferred). If ventilatory assistance is necessary, ventilate gently.
Premedicate	5. Premedicate as appropriate; wait briefly to allow adequate drug effect after administration.
Pharmacologic sedation/anesthesia/ neuromuscular blockade and protection/positioning	6. Administer sedation/anesthesia by IV push. 7. Give neuromuscular blocking agent by IV push. 8. Apply cricoid pressure. 9. Assess for apnea, jaw relaxation, and absence of movement (patient sufficiently relaxed to proceed with intubation).
Placement of endotracheal tube	10. Perform endotracheal intubation. If during intubation oxygen saturation is inadequate, stop laryngoscopy and start ventilation with bag-mask. Monitor pulse oximetry and ensure adequate oxygen saturation. Reattempt intubation. Once intubated, inflate cuff to minimal occlusive volume. Be prepared to place rescue airway if intubation attempts are unsuccessful.
Placement confirmation	11. Confirm placement of endotracheal tube by • direct visualization of ET passing through vocal cords • chest rise/fall with each ventilation (bilateral) • 5-point auscultation: anterior chest L and R, midaxillary line L and R, and over the epigastrium (no breath sounds over epigastrium); look for tube condensation • using end-tidal CO_2 measured by quantitative continuous waveform capnography; if waveform capnography not available, use qualitative exhaled CO_2 detector or esophageal detector device (aspiration technique) • monitoring O_2 saturation (indirect evidence of adequate oxygenation)
Postintubation management	12. Prevent dislodgement: • Secure ET with adhesive/cloth tape or commercial ET holder • Continue cervical spine immobilization • Continue sedation; add paralytics if necessary • Check cuff inflation pressure

Rapid Sequence Intubation

Pharmacologic Agents Used for Rapid Sequence Intubation

Drug	IV/IO Push*	Onset	Duration	Side Effects	Comments
Premedication Agents					
Atropine	0.01-0.02 mg/kg (minimum: 0.1 mg; maximum single dose: 0.5 mg)	1-2 min	2-4 hours	Paradoxical bradycardia can occur with doses <0.1 mg Tachycardia, agitation	Antisialogogue Inhibits bradycardic response to hypoxia, laryngoscopy, and succinylcholine May cause pupil dilation
Glycopyrrolate	0.005-0.01 mg/kg (maximum: 0.2 mg)	1-2 min	4-6 hours	Tachycardia	Antisialogogue Inhibits bradycardic response to hypoxia, laryngoscopy, and succinylcholine
Lidocaine	1-2 mg/kg (maximum: 100 mg)	1-2 min	10-20 min	Myocardial and CNS depression Seizures with high doses	May decrease ICP during RSI May decrease pain on propofol injection

				Sedative/Anesthetic Agents
Etomidate	0.2-0.4 mg/kg Caution: Limit to 1 dose; consider hydrocortisone stress doses for patients in shock	<1 min	5-10 min	Myoclonic activity Inhibition of cortisol synthesis for up to 12 hours	Ultrashort acting No analgesic properties Decreases cerebral metabolic rate and ICP Generally maintains hemodynamic stability Avoid routine use in patients with suspected septic shock
Fentanyl citrate	2-5 mcg/kg	1-3 min	30-60 min	Chest wall rigidity possible with high-dose rapid infusions	Minimum histamine release May lower blood pressure (especially with higher doses or in conjunction with midazolam)
Ketamine	1-2 mg/kg	30-60 sec	10-20 min	Hypertension, tachycardia Increased secretions and laryngospasm Emergence reactions and hallucinations	Dissociative anesthetic agent Limited respiratory depression Bronchodilator May cause myocardial depression in catecholamine-depleted patients Use with caution in patients with potential or increased ICP

Abbreviations: BP, blood pressure; CNS, central nervous system; ICP, intracranial pressure; IO, intraosseous; IV, intravascular.

*Doses provided are guidelines only. Actual dosing may vary depending on patient's clinical status.

(continued)

Pharmacologic Agents Used for Rapid Sequence Intubation (continued)

Drug	IV/IO Push*	Onset	Duration	Side Effects	Comments
Sedative/Anesthetic Agents (continued)					
Midazolam	0.1-0.3 mg/kg (maximum single dose: 10 mg)	2-5 min	15-30 min	Hypotension	Hypotension exacerbated in combination with narcotics and barbiturates No analgesic properties Excellent amnesia
Propofol	1-2 mg/kg	<1 min	5-10 min	Hypotension, especially in patients with inadequate intravascular volume Pain on infusion	No analgesic properties Very short duration of action Less airway reactivity than barbiturates Decreases cerebral metabolic rate and ICP Lidocaine may decrease infusion pain Not recommended in patients with egg/soy allergy
Thiopental	2-5 mg/kg	20-40 sec	5-10 min	Negative inotropic effects Hypotension	Ultrashort-acting barbiturate Decreases cerebral metabolic rate and ICP No analgesic properties

Drug	IV/IO Dose*	Time to Paralysis	Duration of Paralysis	Side Effects	Comments
Neuromuscular Blocking Agents					
Succinylcholine	1-1.5 mg/kg	45-60 sec	5-10 min	Muscle fasciculations May cause rhabdomyolysis; rise in intracranial, intraocular, intragastric pressure; life-threatening hyperkalemia	Depolarizing muscle relaxant Rapid onset, short duration of action Avoid in renal failure, burns, crush injuries after 48 hours, muscular dystrophy and other neuromuscular diseases, hyperkalemia, or family history of malignant hyperthermia Do *not* use to maintain paralysis
Vecuronium	0.1-0.2 mg/kg	1-3 min	45-90 min	Minimal cardiovascular side effects	Nondepolarizing agent The higher the dose, the quicker the onset of action and the longer the duration
Cisatracurium	0.4 mg/kg	2-3 min	90-120 min	Minimal cardiovascular side effects	Nondepolarizing agent Degrades spontaneously, independent of organ elimination
Rocuronium	0.6-1.2 mg/kg	60-90 sec	45-120 min	Minimal cardiovascular side effects	Nondepolarizing agent Rapid onset of action

Abbreviations: ICP, intracranial pressure; IO, intraosseous; IV, intravascular.

*Doses provided are guidelines only. Actual dosing may vary depending on patient's clinical status.

Capnography to Confirm Endotracheal Tube Placement

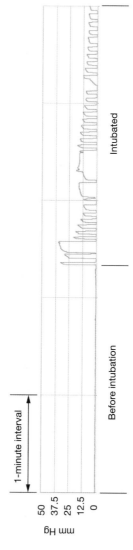

This capnography tracing displays the partial pressure of exhaled carbon dioxide (P_{ETCO_2}) in mm Hg on the vertical axis over time when intubation is performed. Once the patient is intubated, exhaled carbon dioxide is detected, confirming tracheal tube placement. The P_{ETCO_2} varies during the respiratory cycle, with highest values at end-expiration.

Capnography to Monitor Effectiveness of Resuscitation Efforts

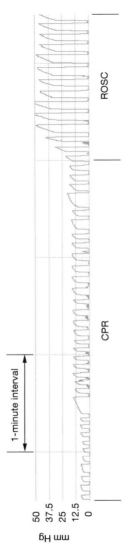

This second capnography tracing displays the $PETCO_2$ in mm Hg on the vertical axis over time. This patient is intubated and receiving CPR. Note that the ventilation rate is approximately 8-10 breaths per minute. Chest compressions are given continuously at a rate of slightly faster than 100/min but are not visible with this tracing. The initial $PETCO_2$ is less than 12.5 mm Hg during the first minute, indicating very low blood flow. The $PETCO_2$ increases to between 12.5 and 25 mm Hg during the second and third minutes, consistent with the increase in blood flow with ongoing resuscitation. Return of spontaneous circulation (ROSC) occurs during the fourth minute. ROSC is recognized by the abrupt increase in the $PETCO_2$ (visible just after the fourth vertical line) to over 40 mm Hg, which is consistent with a substantial improvement in blood flow.

Newborn Resuscitation

Ideally, newborn resuscitation takes place in the delivery room or the neonatal intensive care unit, with trained personnel and appropriate equipment readily available. This form of resuscitation is taught in the **Neonatal Resuscitation Program (NRP)** offered by the American Academy of Pediatrics and the AHA. These pages provide information about initial assessment of the newborn and initial stabilization priorities. *Ensuring adequate ventilation of the baby's lungs is the most important and effective action in neonatal resuscitation.*

Initial Assessment and Stabilization

ABCs of resuscitation	Airway (position and clear if required)
	Breathing (stimulate to breathe)
	Circulation (assess heart rate and color)
Always needed by newborns	Assess baby's risk for requiring resuscitation
	Provide warmth
	Position, clear airway
	Dry, stimulate to breathe
Needed less frequently	Give supplemental oxygen as necessary
	Assist ventilation with positive pressure
	Intubate the trachea
Rarely needed by newborns	Provide chest compressions
	Administer medications

A majority of newborns respond to simple measures. The inverted pyramid reflects relative frequencies of resuscitative efforts for a newborn who does not have meconium-stained amniotic fluid.

Targeted Preductal Spo₂ After Birth

1 min	60%-65%	4 min	75%-80%
2 min	65%-70%	5 min	80%-85%
3 min	70%-75%	10 min	85%-95%

The ranges shown are approximations of the interquartile values reported by Dawson et al (Dawson JA, Kamlin COF, Vento M, Wong C, Cole TJ, Donath SM, Davis PG, Morley CJ. Defining the reference range for oxygen saturation for infants after birth. *Pediatrics*. 2010;125:e1340-e1347) and are adjusted to provide easily remembered targets.

Apgar Score

Sign	0	1	2
Color	Blue or pale	Pink body with blue extremities (acrocyanotic)	Completely pink
Heart rate	Absent	Slow (<100/min)	>100/min
Reflex irritability (to a catheter in the nares, tactile stimulation)	No response	Grimace	Cry or active withdrawal
Muscle tone	Limp	Some flexion	Active motion
Respiration	Absent	Weak cry, hypoventilation	Good, crying

Figure and Apgar Score table reproduced with minor modification from Kattwinkel J, ed. *Textbook of Neonatal Resuscitation*. 5th ed. Elk Grove Village, IL: American Academy of Pediatrics and American Heart Association; 2006.

Overview of Resuscitation in the Delivery Room

Newborn

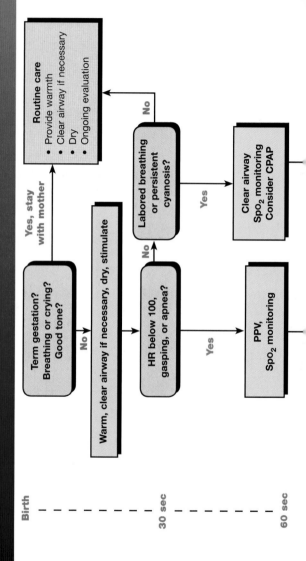

Birth

Term gestation?
Breathing or crying?
Good tone?

Yes, stay with mother →

Routine care
- Provide warmth
- Clear airway if necessary
- Dry
- Ongoing evaluation

No ↓

Warm, clear airway if necessary, dry, stimulate

30 sec

HR below 100, gasping, or apnea?

No →

Labored breathing or persistent cyanosis?

No → Routine care

Yes ↓ (PPV, Spo₂ monitoring)

Yes → **Clear airway**
Spo₂ monitoring
Consider CPAP

60 sec

PPV, Spo₂ monitoring

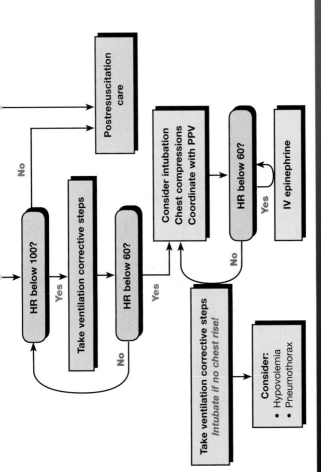

HR below 100?

No → Postresuscitation care

Yes ↓

Take ventilation corrective steps

↓

HR below 60?

No → Postresuscitation care

Yes ↓

Consider intubation
Chest compressions
Coordinate with PPV

←

Take ventilation corrective steps
Intubate if no chest rise!

→

Consider:
• Hypovolemia
• Pneumothorax

↓

HR below 60?

No → (back to Postresuscitation/loop)

Yes ↓ ↻

IV epinephrine

70

Newborn Resuscitation Ratios, Equipment, and Drugs

Initial Cardiopulmonary Resuscitation

Ventilation rate: 40 to 60/min when performed *without* compressions.

Compression rate: 120 events/min (90 compressions interspersed with 30 ventilations).

Compression-ventilation ratio: 3:1 (pause compressions for ventilation).

Medications (epinephrine, volume): Indicated if heart rate remains <60/min despite adequate ventilation with 100% oxygen and chest compressions.

Estimation of Proper Endotracheal Tube Size and Depth of Insertion Based on Infant's Gestational Age and Weight

Weight (g)	Gestational Age (wk)	Laryngoscope Blade	Endotracheal Tube Size (mm)/Catheter Size	Depth of Insertion From Upper Lip (cm)
Below 1000	<28	0	2.5/5F or 6F	6.5-7.0
1000-2000	28-34	0	3.0/6F or 8F	7.0-8.0
2000-3000	34-38	0-1	3.5/8F	8.0-9.0
>3000	>38	1	3.5-4.0/8F	>9.0

Medications Used During or Following Resuscitation of the Newborn

Medications	Dose/Route*	Concentration	Wt (kg)	Total IV/IO Volume (mL)	Precautions
Epinephrine	IV/IO (UVC preferred route) 0.01–0.03 mg/kg Higher IV/IO doses not recommended Endotracheal 0.05–0.1 mg/kg	1:10 000	1 2 3 4	0.1–0.3 0.2–0.6 0.3–0.9 0.4–1.2	Give rapidly. Repeat every 3 to 5 minutes if HR <60 with compressions.
Volume expanders Isotonic crystalloid (normal saline) or blood	10 mL/kg IV/IO		1 2 3 4	10 20 30 40	Indicated for shock. Give over 5 to 10 minutes. Reassess after each bolus.
Special considerations after restoring vital signs:					
Sodium bicarbonate (4.2% solution)	1 to 2 mEq/kg IV/IO	0.5 mEq/mL (4.2% solution)	1 2 3 4	2–4 4–8 6–12 8–16	Only for prolonged resuscitation. Use only if infant is effectively ventilated before administration. Give slow push, minimum 2 minutes.
Dextrose (10% solution)	0.2 g/kg, followed by 5 mL/kg per hour D₁₀ IV/IO infusion	0.1 g/mL	1 2 3 4	2 4 6 8	Indicated for blood glucose <40 mg/dL. Check blood glucose 20 minutes after bolus.

Abbreviations: HR, heart rate; IV/IO, intravenous/intraosseous; UVC, umbilical vein catheter; Wt, weight.

*Endotracheal dose may not result in effective plasma concentration of drug, so vascular access should be established as soon as possible. Drugs given endotracheally require higher dosing than when given IV/IO.

Pediatric Advanced Life Support

Primary cardiac arrest in children is much less common than in adults. **Cardiac arrest in children typically results from progressive deterioration in respiratory or cardiovascular function.** To prevent pediatric cardiac arrest, providers must detect and treat respiratory failure, respiratory arrest, and shock.

Conditions Indicating Need for Rapid Assessment and Potential Cardiopulmonary Support

- Irregular respirations or rate >60 breaths/min
- Heart rate ranges (particularly if associated with poor perfusion)
  - Child ≤2 years of age: <80/min or >180/min
  - Child >2 years of age: <60/min or >160/min
- Poor perfusion, with weak or absent distal pulses
- Increased work of breathing (retractions, nasal flaring, grunting)
- Cyanosis or a decrease in oxyhemoglobin saturation
- Altered level of consciousness (unusual irritability or lethargy or failure to respond to parents or painful procedures)
- Seizures
- Fever with petechiae
- Trauma
- Burns involving >10% of body surface area

Vital Signs in Children

Heart Rate (per minute)*

Age	Awake Rate	Mean	Sleeping Rate
Newborn to 3 months	85 to 205	140	80 to 160
3 months to 2 years	100 to 190	130	75 to 160
2 to 10 years	60 to 140	80	60 to 90
>10 years	60 to 100	75	50 to 90

Respiratory Rate (breaths/min)[†]

Age	Rate
Infant	30 to 60
Toddler	24 to 40
Preschooler	22 to 34
School-aged child	18 to 30
Adolescent	12 to 16

Blood Pressure (BP)[‡]

- Typical systolic BP for 1 to 10 years of age (50th percentile): **90 + (age in years × 2) mm Hg**
- Lower limits of systolic BP for 1 to 10 years of age (5th percentile): **70 + (age in years × 2) mm Hg**
- Lower range of normal systolic BP for >10 years of age: **approximately 90 mm Hg**
- Typical mean arterial pressure (50th percentile): **55 + (age in years × 1.5) mm Hg**

*Modified from Gillette PC, Garson A Jr, Crawford F, Ross B, Ziegler V, Buckles D. Dysrhythmias. In: Adams FH, Emmanouilides GC, Reimenschneider TA, eds. Moss' Heart Disease in Infants, Children, and Adolescents. 4th ed. Baltimore, MD: Williams & Wilkins; 1989:925-939.

[†]Reproduced from Hazinski MF. Children are different. In: Hazinski MF. Manual of Pediatric Critical Care. St Louis, MO: Mosby; 1999:1-13, copyright Elsevier. From Hazinski MF. Children are different. In: Hazinski MF. Nursing Care of the Critically Ill Child. 2nd ed. St Louis, MO: Mosby-Year Book; 1992:1-17, copyright Elsevier.

[‡]Haque IU, Zaritsky AL. Analysis of the evidence for the lower limit of systolic and mean arterial pressure in children. Pediatr Crit Care Med. 2007; 8(2):138-144.

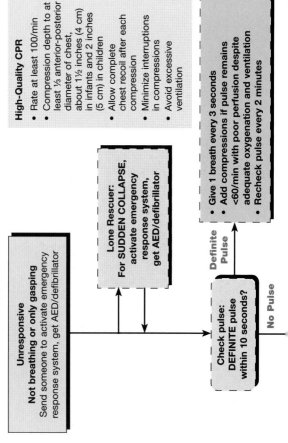

Unresponsive
Not breathing or only gasping
Send someone to activate emergency
response system, get AED/defibrillator

Lone Rescuer:
For SUDDEN COLLAPSE,
activate emergency
response system,
get AED/defibrillator

High-Quality CPR
- Rate at least 100/min
- Compression depth to at least ⅓ anterior-posterior diameter of chest, about 1½ inches (4 cm) in infants and 2 inches (5 cm) in children
- Allow complete chest recoil after each compression
- Minimize interruptions in compressions
- Avoid excessive ventilation

Check pulse: DEFINITE pulse within 10 seconds?

Definite Pulse
- Give 1 breath every 3 seconds
- Add compressions if pulse remains <60/min with poor perfusion despite adequate oxygenation and ventilation
- Recheck pulse every 2 minutes

No Pulse

One Rescuer: Begin cycles of 30 COMPRESSIONS and 2 BREATHS

Two Rescuers: Begin cycles of 15 COMPRESSIONS and 2 BREATHS

After about 2 minutes, activate emergency response system and get AED/defibrillator (if not already done). Use AED as soon as available.

Check rhythm
Shockable rhythm?

Shockable

Give 1 shock
Resume CPR immediately
for 2 minutes

Not Shockable

Resume CPR immediately
for 2 minutes
Check rhythm every 2 minutes; continue until ALS providers take over or victim starts to move

*The boxes bordered with dashed lines are performed by healthcare providers and not by lay rescuers.

73

Pediatric Bradycardia With a Pulse and Poor Perfusion Algorithm

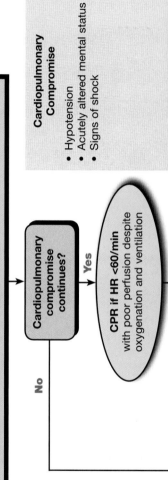

Identify and treat underlying cause

- Maintain patent airway; assist breathing as necessary
- Oxygen
- Cardiac monitor to identify rhythm; monitor blood pressure and oximetry
- IO/IV access
- 12-Lead ECG if available; don't delay therapy

Cardiopulmonary Compromise

- Hypotension
- Acutely altered mental status
- Signs of shock

Cardiopulmonary compromise continues?

No

Yes

CPR if HR <60/min
with poor perfusion despite oxygenation and ventilation

Doses/Details

Epinephrine IO/IV Dose:
0.01 mg/kg (0.1 mL/kg of 1:10 000 concentration).
Repeat every 3-5 minutes.
If IO/IV access not available but endotracheal (ET) tube in place, may give ET dose: 0.1 mg/kg (0.1 mL/kg of 1:1000).

Atropine IO/IV Dose:
0.02 mg/kg. May repeat once. Minimum dose 0.1 mg and maximum single dose 0.5 mg.

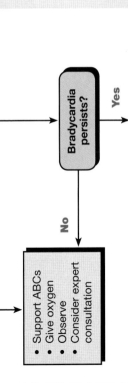

- Support ABCs
- Give oxygen
- Observe
- Consider expert consultation

No

Bradycardia persists?

Yes

- **Epinephrine**
- **Atropine** for increased vagal tone or primary AV block
- Consider transthoracic pacing/transvenous pacing
- Treat underlying causes

If pulseless arrest develops, go to Cardiac Arrest Algorithm

Shout for Help/Activate Emergency Response

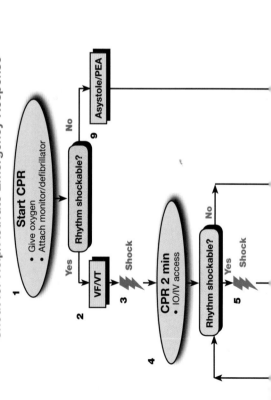

Doses/Details

CPR Quality
- Push hard (≥⅓ of anterior-posterior diameter of chest) and fast (at least 100/min) and allow complete chest recoil
- Minimize interruptions in compressions
- Avoid excessive ventilation
- Rotate compressor every 2 minutes
- If no advanced airway, 15:2 compression-ventilation ratio. If advanced airway, 8-10 breaths per minute with continuous chest compressions

Shock Energy for Defibrillation
First shock 2 J/kg, second shock 4 J/kg, subsequent shocks ≥4 J/kg, maximum 10 J/kg or adult dose.

Drug Therapy
- **Epinephrine IO/IV Dose:**
0.01 mg/kg (0.1 mL/kg of 1:10 000 concentration). Repeat every 3-5 minutes. If no IO/IV access, may give endotracheal dose:
0.1 mg/kg (0.1 mL/kg of 1:1000 concentration).

Algorithm nodes:

1 **Start CPR**
- Give oxygen
- Attach monitor/defibrillator

Rhythm shockable?

Yes →

2 **VF/VT**

3 Shock

4 **CPR 2 min**
- IO/IV access

5 **Rhythm shockable?**

Yes → Shock

No →

9 **Asystole/PEA**

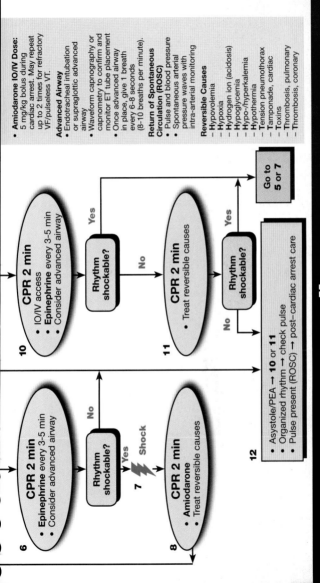

Amiodarone IO/IV Dose:
5 mg/kg bolus during cardiac arrest. May repeat up to 2 times for refractory VF/pulseless VT.

Advanced Airway
- Endotracheal intubation or supraglottic advanced airway
- Waveform capnography or capnometry to confirm and monitor ET tube placement
- Once advanced airway in place, give 1 breath every 6-8 seconds (8-10 breaths per minute).

Return of Spontaneous Circulation (ROSC)
- Pulse and blood pressure
- Spontaneous arterial pressure waves with intra-arterial monitoring

Reversible Causes
- Hypovolemia
- Hypoxia
- Hydrogen ion (acidosis)
- Hypoglycemia
- Hypo-/hyperkalemia
- Hypothermia
- Tension pneumothorax
- Tamponade, cardiac
- Toxins
- Thrombosis, pulmonary
- Thrombosis, coronary

10
- IO/IV access
- **Epinephrine** every 3-5 min
- Consider advanced airway

CPR 2 min

Rhythm shockable? — Yes → Go to **5 or 7**

No

11

CPR 2 min
- Treat reversible causes

Rhythm shockable? — Yes → Go to **5 or 7**

No

6

CPR 2 min
- **Epinephrine** every 3-5 min
- Consider advanced airway

Rhythm shockable? — No

Yes → **Shock** **7**

8

CPR 2 min
- **Amiodarone**
- Treat reversible causes

12
- Asystole/PEA → **10** or **11**
- Organized rhythm → check pulse
- Pulse present (ROSC) → post–cardiac arrest care

75

Pediatric Tachycardia With a Pulse and Poor Perfusion Algorithm

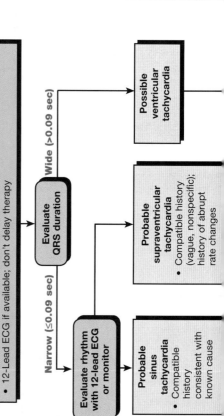

Identify and treat underlying cause

- Maintain patent airway; assist breathing as necessary
- Oxygen
- Cardiac monitor to identify rhythm; monitor blood pressure and oximetry
- IO/IV access
- 12-Lead ECG if available; don't delay therapy

Evaluate QRS duration

Narrow (≤0.09 sec)

Evaluate rhythm with 12-lead ECG or monitor

Probable sinus tachycardia
- Compatible history consistent with known cause

Probable supraventricular tachycardia
- Compatible history (vague, nonspecific); history of abrupt rate changes

Wide (>0.09 sec)

Possible ventricular tachycardia

Doses/Details

Synchronized Cardioversion:
Begin with 0.5-1 J/kg; if not effective, increase to 2 J/kg.
Sedate if needed, but don't delay cardioversion.

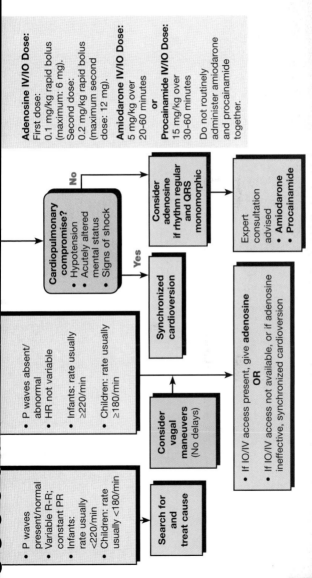

Adenosine IV/IO Dose:
First dose:
0.1 mg/kg rapid bolus
(maximum: 6 mg).
Second dose:
0.2 mg/kg rapid bolus
(maximum second
dose: 12 mg).

Amiodarone IV/IO Dose:
5 mg/kg over
20–60 minutes

or

Procainamide IV/IO Dose:
15 mg/kg over
30–60 minutes

Do not routinely
administer amiodarone
and procainamide
together.

- P waves
  present/normal
- Variable R-R;
  constant PR
- Infants:
  rate usually
  <220/min
- Children: rate
  usually <180/min

**Search for
and treat cause**

- P waves absent/
  abnormal
- HR not variable
- Infants: rate usually
  ≥220/min
- Children: rate usually
  ≥180/min

**Consider
vagal
maneuvers**
(No delays)

- If IO/IV access present, give **adenosine**
  OR
- If IO/IV access not available, or if adenosine
  ineffective, synchronized cardioversion

**Cardiopulmonary
compromise?**
- Hypotension
- Acutely altered
  mental status
- Signs of shock

No → **Consider
adenosine**
if rhythm regular
and QRS monomorphic

Yes → **Synchronized
cardioversion**

Expert
consultation
advised
- **Amiodarone**
- **Procainamide**

76

Pediatric Tachycardia With a Pulse and Adequate Perfusion Algorithm

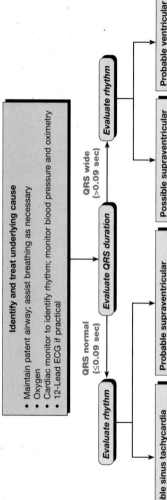

Identify and treat underlying cause
- Maintain patent airway; assist breathing as necessary
- Oxygen
- Cardiac monitor to identify rhythm; monitor blood pressure and oximetry
- 12-Lead ECG if practical

Evaluate QRS duration

QRS normal (≤0.09 sec) — Evaluate rhythm

QRS wide (>0.09 sec) — Evaluate rhythm

Probable sinus tachycardia
- Compatible history consistent with known cause
- P waves present/normal
- Variable R-R with constant PR
- Infants: rate usually <220/min
- Children: rate usually <180/min

Probable supraventricular tachycardia
- Compatible history (vague, nonspecific; history of abrupt rate changes)
- P waves absent/abnormal
- HR not variable with activity
- Infants: rate usually ≥220/min
- Children: rate usually ≥180/min

Possible supraventricular tachycardia (with QRS aberrancy)
- R-R interval regular
- Uniform QRS morphology

Probable ventricular tachycardia

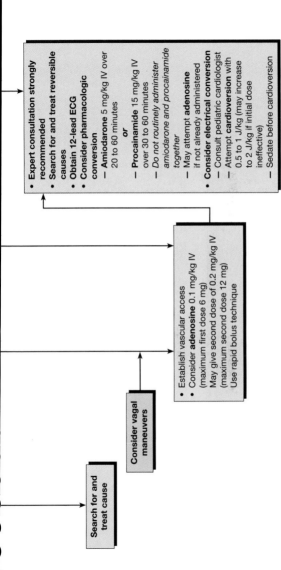

- **Expert consultation strongly recommended**
- Search for and treat reversible causes
- Obtain 12-lead ECG
- Consider pharmacologic conversion
  - **Amiodarone** 5 mg/kg IV over 20 to 60 minutes

    or
  - **Procainamide** 15 mg/kg IV over 30 to 60 minutes
  - *Do not routinely administer amiodarone and procainamide together*
  - May attempt **adenosine** if not already administered
- **Consider electrical conversion**
  - Consult pediatric cardiologist
  - Attempt **cardioversion** with 0.5 to 1 J/kg (may increase to 2 J/kg if initial dose ineffective)
  - Sedate before cardioversion

- Establish vascular access
- Consider **adenosine** 0.1 mg/kg IV (maximum first dose 6 mg)
  May give second dose of 0.2 mg/kg IV (maximum second dose 12 mg)
  Use rapid bolus technique

Consider vagal maneuvers

Search for and treat cause

77

Steps for Pediatric Defibrillation and Cardioversion

Manual Defibrillation (for VF or pulseless VT)

Continue CPR without interruptions during all steps until step 8. Minimize interval from compressions to shock delivery (do not deliver breaths between compressions and shock delivery).

1. Turn on defibrillator.
2. Set *lead switch* to *paddles* (or *lead I, II, or III* if monitor leads are used).
3. Select adhesive pads or paddles. Use the largest pads or paddles that can fit on the patient's chest without touching each other.
4. If using paddles, apply conductive gel or paste. Be sure cables are attached to defibrillator.
5. Position adhesive pads on patient's chest: right anterior chest wall and left axillary positions. If using paddles, apply firm pressure. If patient has an implanted pacemaker, do not position pads/paddles directly over the device. Be sure that oxygen is not directed over patient's chest.

Cardioversion (for unstable SVT or VT with a pulse)

Consider expert consultation for suspected VT.

1. Turn on defibrillator.
2. Set *lead switch* to *paddles* (or *lead I, II, or III* if monitor leads are used).
3. Select adhesive pads to paddles. Use the largest pads or paddles that can fit on the patient's chest without touching each other.
4. If using paddles, apply conductive gel or paste. Be sure cables are attached to defibrillator.
5. Consider sedation.
6. Select *synchronized* mode.
7. Look for markers on R waves indicating that *sync* mode is operative. If necessary, adjust monitor gain until sync markers occur with each R wave.
8. Select energy dose:
   Initial dose: 0.5-1 J/kg
   Subsequent doses: 2 J/kg

6. Select energy dose:

   Initial dose: 2 J/kg (acceptable range 2-4 J/kg)

   Subsequent doses: 4 J/kg or higher (not to exceed 10 J/kg or standard adult dose)

7. Announce "Charging defibrillator," and press *charge* on defibrillator controls or apex paddle.

8. When defibrillator is fully charged, state firm chant, such as

   "I am going to shock on three." Then count.

   "All clear!"

   (Chest compressions should continue until this announcement.)

9. After confirming all personnel are clear of the patient, press the *shock* button on the defibrillator or press the 2 paddle *discharge* buttons simultaneously.

10. Immediately after shock delivery, resume CPR beginning with compressions for 5 cycles (about 2 minutes), and then recheck rhythm. Interruption of CPR should be brief.

9. Announce "Charging defibrillator," and press *charge* on defibrillator controls or apex paddle.

10. When defibrillator is fully charged, state firm chant, such as

    "I am going to shock on three." Then count.

    "All clear!"

11. After confirming all personnel are clear of the patient, press the *shock* button on the defibrillator or press the 2 paddle *discharge* buttons simultaneously. Hold paddles in place until shock is delivered.

12. Check the monitor. If tachycardia persists, increase energy and prepare to cardiovert again.

13. Reset the **sync** mode after each synchronized cardioversion, because most defibrillators default back to unsynchronized mode. This default allows an immediate shock if the cardioversion produces VF.

Note: If VF develops, immediately begin CPR and prepare to deliver an unsynchronized shock (see Manual Defibrillation on left).

78

Considerations for Evaluation of the Cyanotic Neonate

Use this algorithm to determine the likelihood of congenital heart disease (CHD) in the cyanotic neonate.

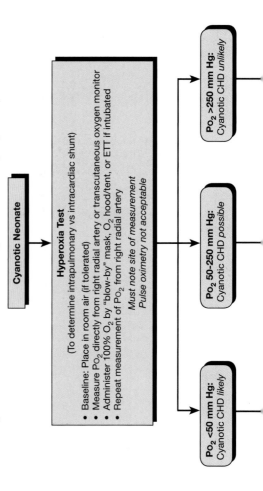

Cyanotic Neonate

Hyperoxia Test
(To determine intrapulmonary vs intracardiac shunt)

- Baseline: Place in room air (if tolerated)
- Measure Po_2 directly from right radial artery or transcutaneous oxygen monitor
- Administer 100% O_2 by "blow-by" mask, O_2 hood/tent, or ETT if intubated
- Repeat measurement of Po_2 from right radial artery

Must note site of measurement
Pulse oximetry not acceptable

Po_2 <50 mm Hg:
Cyanotic CHD *likely*

Po_2 50-250 mm Hg:
Cyanotic CHD *possible*

Po_2 >250 mm Hg:
Cyanotic CHD *unlikely*

- Obtain expert consultation
- Give prostaglandin E$_1$ (PGE$_1$)

- Obtain expert consultation
- Consider PGE$_1$ administration

- Titrate oxygen therapy to avoid hypoxia or hyperoxia
- Avoid hypercarbia

Comparison of Differential and Reverse Differential Cyanosis

(≥10% saturation difference between right arm vs right or left leg)

	Preductal Saturation (eg, right arm)	Postductal Saturation (eg, right or left leg)	Differential Diagnosis	Initial Treatment
Differential Cyanosis	Higher	Lower	• Left-sided obstructive lesion (eg, coarctation of the aorta, interrupted aortic arch, critical aortic stenosis, hypoplastic left heart syndrome) with patent ductus arteriosus • Persistent pulmonary hypertension of the newborn with patent ductus arteriosus	• Administer prostaglandin E$_1$ • Obtain expert consultation
Reverse Differential Cyanosis	Lower	Higher	• Transposition of the great arteries with left-sided obstructive lesion and patent ductus arteriosus • Transposition of the great arteries with persistent pulmonary hypertension of the newborn and patent ductus arteriosus	

Management of Respiratory Emergencies Flowchart

• Airway positioning • Suction as needed • Oxygen • Pulse oximetry • ECG monitor (as indicated) • BLS as indicated

Upper Airway Obstruction
Specific Management for Selected Conditions

Croup	Anaphylaxis	Aspiration Foreign Body
• Nebulized epinephrine • Corticosteroids	• IM epinephrine (or auto-injector) • Albuterol • Antihistamines • Corticosteroids	• Allow position of comfort • Specialty consultation

Lower Airway Obstruction
Specific Management for Selected Conditions

Bronchiolitis	Asthma	
• Nasal suctioning • Bronchodilator trial	• Albuterol ± ipratropium • Corticosteroids • Subcutaneous epinephrine	• Magnesium sulfate • Terbutaline

Lung Tissue (Parenchymal) Disease
Specific Management for Selected Conditions

Pneumonia/Pneumonitis Infectious Chemical Aspiration	Pulmonary Edema Cardiogenic or Noncardiogenic (ARDS)
• Albuterol • Antibiotics (as indicated)	• Consider noninvasive or invasive ventilatory support with PEEP • Consider vasoactive support • Consider diuretic

Disordered Control of Breathing
Specific Management for Selected Conditions

Poisoning/Overdose	Neuromuscular Disease
• Antidote (if available) • Contact poison control	• Consider noninvasive or invasive ventilatory support

Increased ICP	
• Avoid hypoxemia • Avoid hypercarbia • Avoid hyperthermia	

Rapid Sequence Intubation

Pre-event Equipment Checklist for Endotracheal Intubation

☐	Universal precautions (gloves, mask, eye protection)
☐	Cardiac monitor, pulse oximeter, and blood pressure monitoring device
☐	End-tidal CO_2 detector or exhaled CO_2 capnography (or esophageal detector device, if appropriate)
☐	Intravenous and intraosseous infusion equipment
☐	Oxygen supply, bag mask (appropriate size)
☐	Oral/tracheal suction equipment (appropriate size); confirm that it is working
☐	Oral and nasopharyngeal airways (appropriate size)
☐	Endotracheal tubes with stylets (all sizes, with and without cuffs) and sizes 0.5 mm (i.d.) above and below anticipated size for patient
☐	Laryngoscope (curved and straight blades) and/or video laryngoscope; backup laryngoscope available
☐	3-, 5-, and 10-mL syringes to test inflate endotracheal tube balloon
☐	Cuff pressure monitor (if using cuffed tubes)
☐	Adhesive/cloth tape or commercial endotracheal tube holder to secure tube
☐	Towel or pad to align airway by placing under head or torso
☐	Specialty equipment as needed for difficult airway management or anticipated complications (supraglottic, transtracheal, and/or cricothyrotomy)

RSI Protocol for PALS

Pre-event preparation	1. Obtain brief medical history and perform focused physical examination.
	2. Prepare equipment, monitors, personnel, medications.
	3. If neck injury not suspected: place in sniffing position.
	If neck injury suspected: stabilize cervical spine.
Preoxygenate	4. Preoxygenate with FiO_2 of 100% by mask (nonrebreather preferred). If ventilatory assistance is necessary, ventilate gently.
Premedicate/sedate	5. Premedicate and sedate as appropriate; wait briefly to allow adequate sedation after drug administration.
Pharmacologic sedation/anesthesia/ neuromuscular blockade and protection/positioning	6. Administer sedation/anesthesia by IV push.
	7. Give neuromuscular blocking agent by IV push.
	8. Apply cricoid pressure.
	9. Assess for apnea, jaw relaxation, and absence of movement (patient sufficiently relaxed to proceed with intubation).
Placement of endotracheal tube	10. Perform endotracheal intubation. If during intubation oxygen saturation is inadequate, stop laryngoscopy and start ventilation with bag-mask. Monitor pulse oximetry and ensure adequate oxygen saturation. Reattempt intubation. Once intubated, inflate cuff (if cuffed tracheal tube is used) to minimal occlusive volume. Be prepared to place rescue airway if intubation attempts are unsuccessful.
Placement confirmation	11. Confirm placement of endotracheal tube by
	• direct visualization of ET passing through vocal cords
	• chest rise/fall with each ventilation (bilateral)
	• 5-point auscultation: anterior chest L and R, midaxillary line L and R, and over the epigastrium (no breath sounds over epigastrium); look for tube condensation
	• using end-tidal CO_2 detector (or esophageal detector device, if appropriate)
	• monitoring O_2 saturation and exhaled CO_2 levels (capnometry or waveform capnography)
Postintubation management	12. Prevent dislodgement:
	• Secure ET with adhesive/cloth tape or commercial ET holder
	• Continue cervical spine immobilization (if needed)
	• Continue sedation; add paralytics if necessary
	• Check cuff inflation pressure

Pharmacologic Agents Used for Rapid Sequence Intubation in Children

Drug	IV/IO Dose*	Onset	Duration	Side Effects	Comments
Premedication Agents					
Atropine	0.01-0.02 mg/kg (minimum: 0.1 mg; maximum: 0.5 mg)	1-2 min	2-4 hours	Paradoxical bradycardia can occur with doses <0.1 mg Tachycardia, agitation	Antisialogogue Inhibits bradycardic response to hypoxia, laryngoscopy, and succinylcholine May cause pupil dilation
Glycopyrrolate	0.005-0.01 mg/kg (maximum: 0.2 mg)	1-2 min	4-6 hours	Tachycardia	Antisialogogue Inhibits bradycardic response to hypoxia
Lidocaine	1-2 mg/kg	1-2 min	10-20 min	Myocardial and CNS depression with high doses Seizures	May decrease ICP during RSI May decrease pain on propofol injection

Sedative Agents				
Etomidate	0.2-0.4 mg/kg	<1 min	5-10 min	Myoclonic activity Cortisol suppression	Ultrashort acting No analgesic properties Decreases cerebral metabolic rate and ICP Generally maintains hemodynamic stability Avoid routine use in patients with suspected septic shock
Fentanyl citrate	2-5 mcg/kg	1-3 min	30-60 min	Chest wall rigidity possible with high-dose rapid infusions	Minimum histamine release May lower blood pressure (especially with higher doses or in conjunction with midazolam)
Ketamine	1-2 mg/kg	30-60 sec	10-20 min	Hypertension, tachycardia Increased secretions and laryngospasm Emergence reactions/ hallucinations	Dissociative anesthetic agent Limited respiratory depression Bronchodilator May cause myocardial depression in catecholamine-depleted patients Use with caution in patients with potential or increased ICP

Abbreviations: CNS, central nervous system; ICP, intracranial pressure; IO, intraosseous; IV, intravascular; RSI, rapid sequence intubation.

*Doses provided are guidelines only. Actual dosing may vary depending on patient's clinical status.

82

(continued)

Pharmacologic Agents Used for Rapid Sequence Intubation in Children *(continued)*

Drug	IV/IO Dose*	Onset	Duration	Side Effects	Comments
			Sedative Agents *(continued)*		
Midazolam	0.1-0.3 mg/kg (maximum single dose: 10 mg)	2-5 min	15-30 min	Hypotension	Hypotension exacerbated in combination with narcotics and barbiturates No analgesic properties Excellent amnesia
Diazepam	0.2-0.3 mg/kg (maximum single dose: 10 mg)	1-3 min	20-40 min		
Propofol	1-2 mg/kg (up to 3 mg/kg in children 6 months to 5 years of age)	<1 min	5-10 min	Hypotension, especially in patients with inadequate intravascular volume Pain on infusion	No analgesic properties Very short duration of action Less airway reactivity than barbiturates Decreases cerebral metabolic rate and ICP Lidocaine may decrease infusion pain Not recommended in patients with egg/soy allergy
Thiopental	2-5 mg/kg	20-40 sec	5-10 min	Negative inotropic effects Hypotension	Ultrashort-acting barbiturate Decreases cerebral metabolic rate and ICP No analgesic properties

Drug	IV/IO Dose*	Time to Paralysis	Duration of Paralysis	Side Effects	Comments
Neuromuscular Blocking Agents					
Succinylcholine	1-1.5 mg/kg for children; 2 mg/kg for infants	45-60 sec	4-6 min	May cause rhabdomyolysis; rise in intracranial, intraocular, intragastric pressure; life-threatening hyperkalemia	Depolarizing muscle relaxant Rapid onset, short duration of action Avoid in renal failure, burns, crush injuries after 48 hours, muscular dystrophy and other neuromuscular diseases, hyperkalemia, or family history of malignant hyperthermia Do *not* use to maintain paralysis
Vecuronium	0.1-0.3 mg/kg	1-3 min	30-60 min	Minimal cardiovascular side effects	Nondepolarizing agent The higher the dose, the quicker the onset of action and the longer the duration
Rocuronium	0.6-1.2 mg/kg	30-60 sec	30-60 min	Minimal cardiovascular side effects	Nondepolarizing agent Rapid onset of action

Abbreviations: ICP, intracranial pressure; IO, intraosseous; IV, intravascular.

*Doses provided are guidelines only. Actual dosing may vary depending on patient's clinical status.

Septic Shock Algorithm

First hour

Recognize altered mental status and perfusion
Give oxygen and support ventilation; establish vascular access and begin resuscitation according to PALS guidelines
Consider VBG or ABG, lactate, glucose, ionized calcium, cultures, CBC

First hour: Push repeated 20 mL/kg boluses of isotonic crystalloid to treat shock. Give up to 3, 4, or more boluses unless rales, respiratory distress, or hepatomegaly develops.
Additional therapies:
- Correct hypoglycemia and hypocalcemia
- Administer first-dose antibiotics STAT
- Consider ordering STAT vasopressor drip and stress-dose **hydrocortisone***
- Establish second vascular access site if vasoactive infusion anticipated

Fluid responsive (ie, normalized perfu-sion/hemodynamics)?

Yes → Consider ICU monitoring

No →

Begin vasoactive drug therapy and titrate to correct hypotension/poor perfusion; consider establishing arterial and central venous access
- **Normotensive:** Begin **dopamine**
- **Hypotensive vasodilated (warm) shock:** Begin **norepinephrine**
- **Hypotensive vasoconstricted (cold) shock:** Begin **epinephrine** rather than **norepinephrine**

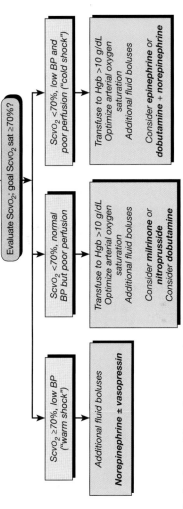

Evaluate ScvO₂; goal ScvO₂ sat ≥70%?

ScvO₂ ≥70%, low BP
("warm shock")

Additional fluid boluses

Norepinephrine ± vasopressin

ScvO₂ <70%, normal
BP but poor perfusion

Transfuse to Hgb >10 g/dL
Optimize arterial oxygen
saturation
Additional fluid boluses

Consider milrinone or
nitroprusside
Consider **dobutamine**

ScvO₂ <70%, low BP and
poor perfusion ("cold shock")

Transfuse to Hgb >10 g/dL
Optimize arterial oxygen
saturation
Additional fluid boluses

Consider **epinephrine** or
dobutamine + norepinephrine

*Fluid-refractory and dopamine- or norepinephrine-dependent shock
defines patient at risk for adrenal insufficiency.

Draw baseline cortisol; consider
ACTH stimulation test if unsure of
need for steroids

If adrenal insufficiency is suspected give
hydrocortisone ~ 2 mg/kg bolus IV; maximum 100 mg

Modified from Brierley J, Carcillo JA, Choong K, Cornell T, Decaen A, Deymann A, Doctor A, Davis A, Duff J, Dugas MA, Duncan A, Evans B, Feldman J, Felmet K, Fisher G, Frankel L, Jeffries H, Greenwald B, Gutierrez J, Hall M, Han YY, Hanson J, Hazelzet J, Herman L, Kiff J, Kissoon N, Kon A, Irazuzta J, Lin J, Lorts A, Mariscalco M, Mehta R, Nadel S, Nguyen T, Nicholson C, Peters M, Okhuysen-Cawley R, Poulton T, Relves M, Rodriguez A, Rozenfeld R, Schnitzler E, Shanley T, Kache S, Skippen P, Torres A, von Dessauer B, Weingarten J, Yeh T, Zaritsky A, Stojadinovic B, Zimmerman J, Zuckerberg A. Clinical practice parameters for hemodynamic support of pediatric and neonatal septic shock: 2007 update from the American College of Critical Care Medicine. *Crit Care Med.* 2009;37(2):666-688.

84

Glasgow Coma Scale* for Adults and Modified Glasgow Coma Scale for Infants and Children†

Response	Adult	Child	Infant	Coded Value
Eye opening	Spontaneous	Spontaneous	Spontaneous	4
	To speech	To speech	To speech	3
	To pain	To pain	To pain	2
	None	None	None	1
Best verbal response	Oriented	Oriented, appropriate	Coos and babbles	5
	Confused	Confused	Irritable, cries	4
	Inappropriate words	Inappropriate words	Cries in response to pain	3
	Incomprehensible sounds	Incomprehensible words or nonspecific sounds	Moans in response to pain	2
	None	None	None	1

Best motor response[‡]	Obeys	Obeys commands	Moves spontaneously and purposely	6
	Localizes	Localizes painful stimulus	Withdraws in response to touch	5
	Withdraws	Withdraws in response to pain	Withdraws in response to pain	4
	Abnormal flexion	Flexion in response to pain	Decorticate posturing (abnormal flexion) in response to pain	3
	Extensor response	Extension in response to pain	Decerebrate posturing (abnormal extension) in response to pain	2
	None	None	None	1
Total score				**3-15**

*Teasdale G, Jennett B. Assessment of coma and impaired consciousness: a practical scale. *Lancet.* 1974;2(7872):81-84.

[†]Modified from Davis RJ, Dean JM, Goldberg AL, Carson BS, Rosenbaum AE, Rogers MC. Head and spinal cord injury. In: Rogers MC, ed. *Textbook of Pediatric Intensive Care.* Baltimore, MD: Williams & Wilkins; 1987:649-699, copyright Lippincott Williams & Wilkins; James HE, Trauner DA. The Glasgow Coma Scale. In: James HE, Anas NG, Perkin RM, eds. *Brain Insults in Infants and Children: Pathophysiology and Management.* Orlando, FL: Grune & Stratton; 1985:179-182; Jennett B, Teasdale G, Braakman R, Minderhoud J, Knill-Jones R. Predicting outcome in individual patients after severe head injury. *Lancet.* 1976;1:1031-1034; Morray JP, Tyler DC, Jones TK, Stuntz JT, Lemire RJ. Coma scale for use in brain-injured children. *Crit Care Med.* 1984;12:1018-1020; and Hazinski MF. Neurologic disorders. In: Hazinski MF. *Nursing Care of the Critically Ill Child.* 2nd ed. St Louis, MO: Mosby-Year Book; 1992:521-628, copyright Elsevier.

[‡]If the patient is intubated, unconscious, or preverbal, the most important part of this scale is motor response. Providers should carefully evaluate this component.

Field Triage of the Injured Patient

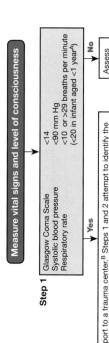

Measure vital signs and level of consciousness

Step 1

Glasgow Coma Scale <14
Systolic blood pressure <90 mm Hg
Respiratory rate <10 or >29 breaths per minute
(<20 in infant aged <1 year[A])

Yes → Transport to a trauma center.[B] Steps 1 and 2 attempt to identify the most seriously injured patients. These patients should be transported preferentially to the highest level of care in the trauma system.

No → Assess anatomy of injury.

Step 2[C]

- All penetrating injuries to head, neck, torso, and extremities proximal to elbow and knee
- Flail chest
- Two or more proximal long-bone fractures
- Crushed, degloved, or mangled extremity
- Amputation proximal to wrist and ankle
- Pelvic fractures
- Open or depressed skull fracture
- Paralysis

Yes → Transport to a trauma center. Steps 1 and 2 attempt to identify the most seriously injured patients. These patients should be transported preferentially to the highest level of care in the trauma system.

No → Assess mechanism of injury and evidence of high-energy impact.

From Sasser SM, Hunt RC, Sullivent EE, Wald MM, Mitchko J, Jurkovich GJ, Henry MC, Salomone JP, Wang SC, Galli RL, Cooper A, Brown LH, Sattin RW; National Expert Panel on Field Triage, Centers for Disease Control and Prevention. Guidelines for field triage of injured patients: recommendations of the National Expert Panel on Field Triage. *MMWR Recomm Rep.* 2009;58:1-35. Adapted from Committee on Trauma, American College of Surgeons. *Resources for Optimal Care of the Injured Patient.* Chicago, IL: American College of Surgeons; 2006. Footnotes have been added to enhance understanding of field triage by persons outside the acute injury care field.

[A] The upper limit of respiratory rate in infants is >29 breaths per minute to maintain a higher level of overtriage for infants.

[B] Trauma centers are designated level I-IV, with level I representing the highest level of trauma care available.

[C] Any injury noted in steps 2 and 3 triggers a "yes" response.

Step 3[C]

- Falls
  - Adults: >20 feet (1 story = 10 feet)
  - Children[D]: >10 feet or 2 or 3 times the height of the child
- High-risk motor vehicle crash
  - Intrusion[E]: >12 inches occupant site; >18 inches any site
  - Ejection (partial or complete) from automobile
  - Death in same passenger compartment
  - Vehicle telemetry data consistent with high-risk injury
- Motor vehicle vs pedestrian/bicyclist thrown, run over, or with significant (>20 mph) impact[F]
- Motorcycle crash >20 mph

Yes → Transport to closest appropriate trauma center, which, depending on the trauma system, needs not be the highest-level trauma center.[G] → Assess special patient or system considerations.

No → Assess special patient or system considerations.

Step 4

- Age
  - Older adults[H]: Risk of injury/death increases after age 55 years
  - Children: Should be triaged preferentially to pediatric-capable trauma centers
- Anticoagulation and bleeding disorders
- Burns
  - Without other trauma mechanism: triage to burn facility[I]
  - With trauma mechanism: triage to trauma center[I]
- Time-sensitive extremity injury[J]
- End-stage renal disease requiring dialysis
- Pregnancy >20 weeks
- EMS[K] provider judgment

Yes → Contact medical control and consider transport to a trauma center of a specific resource hospital.

No → Transport according to protocol.[L]

When in doubt, transport to a trauma center

[D] Age <15 years.

[E] Intrusion refers to interior compartment intrusion, as opposed to deformation, which refers to exterior damage.

[F] Includes pedestrians or bicyclists thrown or run over by a motor vehicle or those with estimated impact >20 mph with a motor vehicle.

[G] Local or regional protocols should be used to determine the most appropriate level of trauma center; an appropriate center need not be level I.

[H] Age >55 years.

[I] Patients with both burns and concomitant trauma for whom the burn injury poses the greatest risk for morbidity and mortality should be transferred to a burn center. If the nonburn trauma presents a greater immediate risk, the patient may be stabilized in a trauma center and then transferred to a burn center.

[J] Injuries such as an open fracture or fracture with neurovascular compromise.

[K] Emergency medical services.

[L] Patients who do not meet any of the triage criteria in steps 1-4 should be transported to the most appropriate medical facility as outlined in local EMS protocols.

Systemic Responses to Blood Loss in Pediatric Patients

System	Mild Blood Volume Loss (<30%)	Moderate Blood Volume Loss (30%-45%)	Severe Blood Volume Loss (>45%)
Cardiovascular	Increased heart rate; weak, thready peripheral pulses; normal systolic blood pressure (80-90 + 2 × age in years); normal pulse pressure	Markedly increased heart rate; weak, thready central pulses; absent peripheral pulses; low normal systolic blood pressure (70-80 + 2 × age in years); narrowed pulse pressure	Tachycardia followed by bradycardia; very weak or absent peripheral pulses; hypotension (<70 + 2 × age in years); undetectable diastolic blood pressure (or widened pulse pressure)
Central nervous system	Anxious; irritable; confused	Lethargic; dulled response to pain*	Comatose
Skin	Cool, mottled; prolonged capillary refill	Cyanotic; markedly prolonged capillary refill	Pale and cold
Urine output†	Low to very low	Minimal	None

*The child's dulled response to pain with this degree of blood loss (30%-45%) may be indicated by a decreased response to IV catheter insertion.
†After initial decompression by urinary catheter. Low normal is 2 mL/kg per hour (infant), 1.5 mL/kg per hour (younger child), 1 mL/kg per hour (older child), and 0.5 mL/kg per hour (adolescent). Intravenous contrast can falsely elevate urinary output.
Modified from American College of Surgeons Committee on Trauma. *Advanced Trauma Life Support® for Doctors: ATLS Student Course Manual.* 8th ed. Chicago, IL: American College of Surgeons; 2008.

Approach to the Child With Multiple Injuries

Effective trauma resuscitation requires a team effort. The assessments and interventions below may be performed simultaneously. Initiate CPR when needed.

1. Before arrival, notify trauma surgeon with pediatric expertise.

2. Open airway with jaw thrust, maintaining manual cervical spine stabilization.

3. Clear the oropharynx with a rigid suction device; assess breathing.

4. Administer 100% oxygen by nonrebreathing mask if child is responsive and breathing spontaneously.

5. Ventilate with bag-mask device and 100% oxygen if child has inadequate respiratory effort or respiratory distress or is unresponsive. Hyperventilate only if there are signs of impending brain herniation.

6. Provide advanced airway management with appropriate manual cervical spine stabilization if the child has signs of respiratory failure or is unresponsive. Trained healthcare providers may attempt endotracheal intubation; confirm endotracheal tube placement with clinical assessment and a device (eg, exhaled CO_2 detector, esophageal detector device). If the child is unconscious during bag-mask ventilation, consider use of an oropharyngeal airway and cricoid pressure.

Approach to Fluid Resuscitation in Child With Multiple Injuries

Signs of inadequate systemic perfusion are present*

↓

Rapid infusion (<20 minutes) 20 mL/kg of LR or NS†

↓

Continued signs of inadequate systemic perfusion?

Yes

↓

Second rapid infusion 20 mL/kg of LR or NS†

Continued signs of inadequate systemic perfusion?

Yes

- Third rapid infusion 20 mL/kg of LR or NS†

  or

- Packed RBCs (10 mL/kg), mixed with NS, bolus

  Repeat every 20 to 30 minutes, as needed

---

*In child with severe trauma and life-threatening blood loss:
  - Blood for STAT type and crossmatch; type-specific blood is preferred, time permitting
  - Use O-negative blood in females and O-positive or O-negative blood in males when possible.

†If LR is not available, NS may be used.

---

7. While maintaining airway patency and spine stabilization, assess signs of circulation.

8. Control external bleeding with direct pressure if indicated.

9. Treat tension pneumothorax via needle decompression.

10. Establish vascular access; obtain blood samples for blood type and crossmatch studies.

11. Rapidly infuse 20 mL/kg isotonic crystalloid for inadequate perfusion.

12. Immobilize the neck with a semirigid collar, head immobilizer, and tape. In prehospital settings, immobilize thighs, pelvis, shoulders, and head to long spine board.

13. Consider gastric decompression (an orogastric tube is preferred if head trauma is present).

14. Infuse a second isotonic crystalloid bolus if signs of shock are present. Consider blood products for major hemorrhage.

15. Consider need for surgical exploration if hypotension is present on arrival or if hemodynamic instability persists despite crystalloid and blood administration.

Estimation of Maintenance Fluid Requirements

- **Infants <10 kg:** 4 mL/kg per hour

  Example: For an 8-kg infant, estimated maintenance fluid rate

  = 4 mL/kg per hour × 8 kg

  = 32 mL per hour

- **Children 10-20 kg:** 4 mL/kg per hour for the first 10 kg + 2 mL/kg per hour for each kg above 10 kg

  Example: For a 15-kg child, estimated maintenance fluid rate

  = (4 mL/kg per hour × 10 kg)
  + (2 mL/kg per hour × 5 kg)

  = 40 mL/hour + 10 mL/hour

  = 50 mL/hour

Management of Shock After ROSC

Optimize Ventilation and Oxygenation

- Titrate FIO_2 to maintain oxyhemoglobin saturation 94%-99%; if possible, wean FIO_2 if saturation is 100%
- Consider advanced airway placement and waveform capnography

Assess for and Treat Persistent Shock

- Identify, treat contributing factors.*
- Consider 20 mL/kg IV/IO boluses of isotonic crystalloid. Consider smaller boluses (eg, 10 mL/kg) if poor cardiac function suspected.
- Consider the need for inotropic and/or vasopressor support for fluid-refractory shock.

*Possible Contributing Factors

Hypovolemia
Hypoxia
Hydrogen ion (acidosis)
Hypoglycemia
Hypo-/hyperkalemia
Hypothermia
Tension pneumothorax
Tamponade, cardiac
Toxins
Thrombosis, pulmonary
Thrombosis, coronary
Trauma

- **Children >20 kg:** 4 mL/kg per hour for the first 10 kg + 2 mL/kg per hour for kg 11-20 + 1 mL/kg per hour for each kg above 20 kg.

Example: For a 28-kg child, estimated maintenance fluid rate

$$= (4 \text{ mL/kg per hour} \times 10 \text{ kg})$$
$$+ (2 \text{ mL/kg per hour} \times 10 \text{ kg})$$
$$+ (1 \text{ mL/kg per hour} \times 8 \text{ kg})$$
$$= 40 \text{ mL per hour} + 20 \text{ mL per hour}$$
$$+ 8 \text{ mL per hour}$$
$$= 68 \text{ mL per hour}$$

Following initial stabilization, adjust the rate and composition of intravenous fluids based on the patient's clinical condition and state of hydration. In general, provide a continuous infusion of a dextrose-containing solution for infants. Avoid hypotonic solutions in critically ill children; for most patients use isotonic fluid such as normal saline (0.9% NaCl) or lactated Ringer's solution with or without dextrose, based on the child's clinical status.

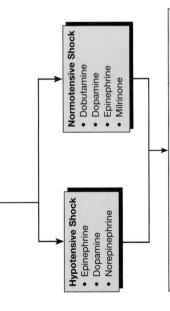

Hypotensive Shock
- Epinephrine
- Dopamine
- Norepinephrine

Normotensive Shock
- Dobutamine
- Dopamine
- Epinephrine
- Milrinone

- Monitor for and treat agitation and seizures
- Monitor for and treat hypoglycemia
- Assess blood gas, serum electrolytes, calcium
- If patient remains comatose after resuscitation from cardiac arrest, consider therapeutic hypothermia (32°C-34°C)
- Consider consultation and patient transport to tertiary care center

Pediatric Resuscitation Supplies
Based on Color-Coded Resuscitation Tape

Equipment	GRAY 3-5 kg	PINK Small Infant 6-7 kg	RED Infant 8-9 kg	PURPLE Toddler 10-11 kg	YELLOW Small Child 12-14 kg	WHITE Child 15-18 kg	BLUE Child 19-23 kg	ORANGE Large Child 24-29 kg	GREEN Adult 30-36 kg
Resuscitation bag		Infant/child	Infant/child	Child	Child	Child	Child	Child	Adult
Oxygen mask (NRB)		Pediatric	Pediatric	Pediatric	Pediatric	Pediatric	Pediatric	Pediatric	Pediatric/adult
Oral airway (mm)		50	50	60	60	60	70	80	80
Laryngoscope blade (size)		1 Straight	1 Straight	1 Straight	2 Straight	2 Straight	2 Straight or curved	2 Straight or curved	3 Straight or curved
ET tube (mm)†		3.5 Uncuffed 3.0 Cuffed	3.5 Uncuffed 3.0 Cuffed	4.0 Uncuffed 3.5 Cuffed	4.5 Uncuffed 4.0 Cuffed	5.0 Uncuffed 4.5 Cuffed	5.5 Uncuffed 5.0 Cuffed	6.0 Cuffed	6.5 Cuffed
ET tube insertion length (cm)	3 kg 9-9.5 4 kg 9.5-10 5 kg 10-10.5	10.5-11	10.5-11	11-12	13.5	14-15	16.5	17-18	18.5-19.5
Suction catheter (F)		8	8	10	10	10	10	10	10-12
BP cuff	Neonatal #5/infant	Infant/child	Infant/child	Child	Child	Child	Child	Child	Small adult
IV catheter (ga)		22-24	22-24	20-24	18-22	18-22	18-20	18-20	16-20
IO (ga)		18/15	18/15	15	15	15	15	15	15
NG tube (F)		5-8	5-8	8-10	10	10	12-14	14-18	16-18
Urinary catheter (F)	5	8	8	8-10	10	10-12	10-12	12	12
Chest tube (F)		10-12	10-12	16-20	20-24	20-24	24-32	28-32	32-38

Abbreviations: BP, blood pressure; ET, endotracheal; F, French; IO, intraosseous; IV, intravenous; NG, nasogastric; NRB, nonbreathing.

*For Gray column, use Pink or Red equipment sizes if no size is listed.

†Per 2005 AHA Guidelines, in the hospital cuffed or uncuffed tubes may be used (see below for sizing of cuffed tubes).

Adapted from Broselow™ Pediatric Emergency Tape. Distributed by Armstrong Medical Industries, Lincolnshire, IL. Copyright 2007 Vital Signs, Inc. All rights reserved.

Estimating Endotracheal Tube Size and Depth of Insertion

Tube Size

Several formulas, such as the ones below, allow estimation of proper endotracheal tube size (internal diameter [i.d.]) for children 2 to 10 years of age, based on the child's age:

Uncuffed endotracheal tube size (mm i.d.) = (age in years/4) + 4

During preparation for intubation, providers also should have ready at the bedside uncuffed endotracheal tubes 0.5 mm smaller and larger than that estimated from the above formula.

The formula for estimation of a cuffed endotracheal tube size is as follows:

Cuffed endotracheal tube size (mm i.d.) = (age in years/4) + 3.5

Typical cuffed inflation pressure should be <20 to 25 cm H_2O.

Depth of Insertion

The formula for estimation of depth of insertion (measured at the lip) can be estimated from the child's age or the tube size.

Depth of insertion (cm) for children >2 years of age = (age in years/2) + 12

or

Depth of insertion = tube i.d. (mm) × 3

Confirm placement with both clinical assessment (eg, breath sounds, chest expansion) and device (eg, exhaled CO_2 detector). Watch for marker on endotracheal tube at vocal cords.

Administration Notes

Peripheral Intravenous (IV):	Resuscitation drugs administered via peripheral IV catheter should be followed by a bolus of at least 5 mL NS to move drug into central circulation.
Intraosseous (IO):	Drugs that can be administered by IV route may be administered by IO route. They should be followed by a bolus of at least 5 mL NS to move drug into central circulation.
Endotracheal:	IV/IO administration is preferred because it provides more reliable drug delivery and pharmacologic effect. Drugs that can be administered by endotracheal route are noted in the tables below. Optimal endotracheal doses have not yet been established. Doses given by ET route should generally be higher than standard IV doses. For infants and children, dilute the medication with NS to a volume of 3 to 5 mL, instill in the endotracheal tube, and follow with flush of 3 to 5 mL. Provide 5 positive-pressure breaths after medication is instilled.
Formula for verification of dose and continuous infusion rate:	$$\text{Infusion rate (mL/h)} = \frac{\text{Weight (kg)} \times \text{dose (mcg/kg per minute)} \times 60 \text{ min/h}}{\text{Concentration (mcg/mL)}}$$

Drug/Therapy	Indications/Precautions	Pediatric Dosage
Adenosine	**Indications** Drug of choice for treatment of symptomatic SVT. **Precautions** • Very short half-life. • Limited adult data suggest need to reduce dose in patients taking carbamazepine and dipyridamole. • Less effective (larger doses may be required) in patients taking theophylline or caffeine.	**IV/IO Administration** • First dose: – 0.1 mg/kg IV/IO *rapid* push. – Maximum dose: 6 mg. • Second dose: – 0.2 mg/kg IV/IO *rapid* push. – Maximum dose: 12 mg. • Follow immediately with 5 to 10 mL NS flush. • Continuous ECG monitoring. **Injection Technique** • Record rhythm strip during administration. • Draw up adenosine dose and flush (5 to 10 mL) in 2 separate syringes. • Attach both syringes to IV injection port closest to patient. • Clamp IV tubing above injection port. • Push IV adenosine as *quickly* as possible (1 to 3 seconds). • While maintaining pressure on adenosine plunger, push NS flush as *rapidly as possible* after adenosine. • Unclamp IV tubing.

Pediatric Advanced Life Support Drugs

Drug/Therapy	Indications/Precautions	Pediatric Dosage
Albuterol Nebulized solution: 0.5% (5 mg/mL) Prediluted nebulized solution: 0.63 mg/3 mL NS, 1.25 mg/3 mL NS, 2.5 mg/3 mL NS (0.083%) MDI: 90 mcg/puff	**Indications** Bronchodilator, β_2-adrenergic agent • Asthma. • Anaphylaxis (bronchospasm). • Hyperkalemia.	**For Asthma, Anaphylaxis (Mild to Moderate), Hyperkalemia** • **MDI (every 20 minutes)** — 4 to 8 puffs (inhalation) PRN with spacer. • **Nebulizer (every 20 minutes)** — Weight <20 kg: 2.5 mg/dose (inhalation). — Weight >20 kg: 5 mg/dose (inhalation). **For Asthma, Anaphylaxis (Severe)** • **Continuous nebulizer** — 0.5 mg/kg per hour continuous inhalation (maximum dose 20 mg/h). • **MDI** (recommended if intubated) — 4 to 8 puffs (inhalation) via endotracheal tube every 20 minutes PRN or with spacer if not intubated.
Alprostadil (PGE$_1$) (See *Prostaglandin E$_1$*)		

Amiodarone

Indications

Can be used for treatment of atrial and ventricular arrhythmias in children, particularly ectopic atrial tachycardia, junctional ectopic tachycardia, and ventricular tachycardia/ventricular fibrillation.

Precautions

- May produce hypotension. May prolong QT interval and increase propensity for polymorphic ventricular arrhythmias. Therefore, routine administration in combination with procainamide is not recommended without expert consultation.

- Use with caution if hepatic failure is present.

- Terminal elimination is extremely long (elimination half-life with long-term oral dosing is up to 40 days).

For Refractory VF, Pulseless VT

5 mg/kg IV/IO bolus; can repeat the 5 mg/kg IV/IO bolus up to total dose of 15 mg/kg (2.2 g in adolescents) IV per 24 hours.

Maximum single dose: 300 mg.

For Perfusing Supraventricular and Ventricular Arrhythmias

Loading dose: 5 mg/kg IV/IO over 20 to 60 minutes (maximum single dose: 300 mg). Can repeat to maximum of 15 mg/kg (2.2 g in adolescents) per day IV.

Pediatric Advanced Life Support Drugs

Drug/Therapy	Indications/Precautions	Pediatric Dosage
Atropine Sulfate Can be given by endotracheal tube	**Indications** • Symptomatic bradycardia (usually secondary to vagal stimulation). • Toxins/overdose (eg, organophosphate, carbamate). • Rapid sequence intubation (RSI): ie, age <1 year, age 1 to 5 years receiving succinylcholine, age >5 years receiving second dose of succinylcholine. **Precautions** • Contraindicated in angle-closure glaucoma, tachyarrhythmias, thyrotoxicosis. • Drug blocks bradycardic response to hypoxia. Monitor with pulse oximetry.	**Symptomatic Bradycardia** • **IV/IO:** 0.02 mg/kg (minimum dose: 0.1 mg). — Maximum single dose: 0.5 mg. — May repeat dose once. — Maximum total dose for child: 1 mg; for adolescent: 3 mg. — Larger doses may be needed for organophosphate poisoning. • **ET:** 0.04 to 0.06 mg/kg. **Toxins/Overdose** • <12 years: 0.02 to 0.05 mg/kg IV/IO initially, then repeated IV/IO every 20 to 30 minutes until muscarinic symptoms reverse. • >12 years: 2 mg IV/IO initially, then 1 to 2 mg IV/IO every 20 to 30 minutes until muscarinic symptoms reverse. **RSI** • **IV/IO:** 0.01 to 0.02 mg/kg (minimum dose: 0.1 mg; maximum dose: 0.5 mg). • **IM:** 0.02 mg/kg.

Calcium Chloride

10% = 100 mg/mL =
27.2 mg/mL elemental
calcium

Indications

- Treatment of documented or suspected conditions:
  - Hypocalcemia.
  - Hyperkalemia.
- Consider for treatment of:
  - Hypermagnesemia.
  - Calcium channel blocker overdose.

Precautions

- Do not use routinely during resuscitation (may contribute to cellular injury).
- Not recommended for routine treatment of asystole or PEA.
- Rapid IV administration may cause hypotension, bradycardia, or asystole (particularly if patient is receiving digoxin).
- Do not mix with or infuse immediately before or after sodium bicarbonate without intervening flush.

IV/IO Administration

- 20 mg/kg (0.2 mL/kg) slow IV/IO push.
- May repeat if documented or suspected clinical indication persists (eg, toxicologic problem).
- Central venous administration preferred if available.

93

Pediatric Advanced Life Support Drugs

Drug/Therapy	Indications/Precautions	Pediatric Dosage

Calcium Gluconate
 	
10% = 100 mg/mL = 9 mg/mL elemental calcium
	Indications
	• Treatment of documented or suspected conditions:
	  – Hypocalcemia.
	  – Hyperkalemia.
	• Consider for treatment of:
	  – Hypermagnesemia.
	  – Calcium channel blocker overdose.
	
	Precautions
	• Do not use routinely during resuscitation (may contribute to cellular injury).
	• Not recommended for routine treatment of asystole or PEA.
	• Rapid IV administration may cause hypotension, bradycardia, or asystole (particularly if patient is receiving digoxin).
	• Do not mix with or infuse immediately before or after sodium bicarbonate without intervening flush.
		IV/IO Administration
		• 60 to 100 mg/kg (0.6 to 1 mL/kg) slow IV/IO push.
		• May repeat if documented or suspected clinical indication persists (eg, toxicologic problem).
		• Central venous administration preferred if available.

Corticosteroids

Precautions
May cause hypertension, hyperglycemia, and increased risk of gastric bleeding.

Dexamethasone

Indications
- Croup.
- Asthma.

For Croup
- 0.6 mg/kg PO/IM/IV × 1 dose (maximum dose: 16 mg).

For Asthma
- 0.6 mg/kg PO/IM/IV every 24 hours (maximum dose: 16 mg).

Hydrocortisone

Indications
Treatment of adrenal insufficiency (may be associated with septic shock).

Adrenal Insufficiency
2 mg/kg IV/IO bolus (maximum dose: 100 mg).

Methylprednisolone

Indications
- Asthma (status asthmaticus).
- Anaphylactic shock.

(Use sodium succinate salt)

Status Asthmaticus, Anaphylactic Shock
- Load: 2 mg/kg IV/IO/IM (maximum: 60 mg).
- Maintenance: 0.5 mg/kg IV every 6 hours or 1 mg/kg every 12 hours up to 120 mg/day.

Pediatric Advanced Life Support Drugs

Drug/Therapy	Indications/Precautions	Pediatric Dosage
Dobutamine	**Indications** Treatment of shock associated with high systemic vascular resistance (eg, congestive heart failure or cardiogenic shock). Ensure adequate intravascular volume. **Precautions** • May produce or exacerbate hypotension. • May produce tachyarrhythmias. • Do not mix with sodium bicarbonate. • Extravasation may cause tissue injury.	**Continuous IV/IO Infusion** • Titrate to desired effect. Typical infusion dose: 2 to 20 mcg/kg per minute.

Dopamine

Indications
Treatment of shock with adequate intra-vascular volume and stable rhythm.

Precautions
- High infusion rates (>20 mcg/kg per minute) may cause splanchnic vasoconstriction, ischemia.
- May produce tachyarrhythmias.
- Do not mix with sodium bicarbonate.
- Extravasation may cause tissue injury.
- May affect thyroid function.

Continuous IV/IO Infusion
- Titrate to desired effect. Typical infusion dose: 2 to 20 mcg/kg per minute.

Note: If infusion dose >20 mcg/kg per minute is required, consider using alternative adrenergic agent (eg, epinephrine/norepinephrine).

Pediatric Advanced Life Support Drugs

Drug/Therapy	Indications/Precautions	Pediatric Dosage
Epinephrine Standard: 1:10 000 or 0.1 mg/mL High: 1:1000 or 1 mg/mL Can be given via endotracheal tube	**Indications** • Bolus IV therapy — Treatment of pulseless arrest. — Treatment of symptomatic bradycardia unresponsive to O_2 and ventilation. • Continuous IV infusion — Shock (poor perfusion) or hypotension in patient with adequate intravascular volume and stable rhythm. — Clinically significant bradycardia. — β-Blocker or calcium channel blocker overdose. — Pulseless arrest when bolus therapy fails. • IM bolus therapy — Anaphylaxis. — Severe status asthmaticus.	**Pulseless Arrest** • **IV/IO dose:** 0.01 mg/kg (0.1 mL/kg of 1:10 000 standard concentration). Administer every 3 to 5 minutes during arrest (maximum dose: 1 mg). • **All endotracheal doses:** 0.1 mg/kg (0.1 mL/kg of 1:1000 high concentration). — Administer every 3 to 5 minutes of arrest until IV/IO access achieved; then begin with first IV dose. **Symptomatic Bradycardia** • **All IV/IO doses:** 0.01 mg/kg (0.1 mL/kg of 1:10 000 standard concentration). • **All endotracheal doses:** 0.1 mg/kg (0.1 mL/kg of 1:1000 high concentration).

(continued)

Epinephrine
(continued)

Precautions
- May produce tachyarrhythmias.
- High-dose infusions may produce vasoconstriction, may compromise perfusion; low doses may decrease renal and splanchnic blood flow.
- Do not mix with sodium bicarbonate.
- Correct hypoxemia.
- Contraindicated in treatment of VT secondary to cocaine (may be considered if VF develops).

Continuous IV/IO Infusion
Once tubing is primed, titrate to response. Typical initial infusion: 0.1 to 1 mcg/kg per minute. Higher doses may be effective.

Anaphylaxis/Severe Status Asthmaticus
- IM dose: 0.01 mg/kg (0.01 mL/kg of 1:1000 high concentration).
- Maximum single dose: 0.3 mg.
- Repeat as needed.

Pediatric Advanced Life Support Drugs

Drug/Therapy	Indications/Precautions	Pediatric Dosage
Etomidate	**Indications** • Ultrashort-acting nonbarbiturate, non-benzodiazepine sedative-hypnotic agent with no analgesic properties. • Produces rapid sedation with minimal cardiovascular or respiratory depression. • Sedative of choice for hypotensive patients. • Decreases ICP, cerebral blood flow, and cerebral basal metabolic rate. **Precautions** • May suppress cortisol production after a single dose. Consider administration of stress dose hydrocortisone (2 mg/kg; maximum dose 100 mg). • Avoid routine use in septic shock. • May also cause myoclonic activity (coughing, hiccups) and may exacerbate focal seizure disorders. • Relative contraindications include known adrenal insufficiency or history of focal seizure disorder.	**For Rapid Sedation** • IV/IO dose of 0.2 to 0.4 mg/kg infused over 30 to 60 seconds will produce rapid sedation that lasts 10 to 15 minutes. • Maximum dose: 20 mg.

Glucose

Indications

Treatment of hypoglycemia (documented or strongly suspected).

Precautions

- Use bedside glucose test to confirm hypoglycemia; hyperglycemia may worsen neurologic outcome of cardiopulmonary arrest or trauma; do not administer routinely during resuscitation.
- Maximum concentration for newborn administration: 12.5% (0.125 g/mL).

IV/IO Infusion

0.5 to 1 g/kg (maximum recommended IV/IO concentration: 25%; can prepare by mixing 50% dextrose 1:1 with sterile water).
- **50%** dextrose (0.5 g/mL); give 1 to 2 mL/kg.
- **25%** dextrose (0.25 g/mL); give 2 to 4 mL/kg.
- **10%** dextrose (0.1 g/mL); give 5 to 10 mL/kg.
- **5%** dextrose (0.05 g/mL); give 10 to 20 mL/kg if volume tolerated.

Inamrinone
(Aminone)

Indications

Myocardial dysfunction and increased systemic or pulmonary vascular resistance, including
- Congestive heart failure in postoperative cardiovascular surgical patients.
- Shock with high systemic vascular resistance.

Precautions

- May produce hypotension, particularly in volume-depleted patients.
- Long elimination half-life.
- May cause thrombocytopenia.
- Drug may accumulate in renal failure and in patients with low cardiac output.

Loading Dose

0.75 to 1 mg/kg IV/IO over 5 minutes; may repeat twice (maximum: 3 mg/kg).

Continuous Infusion

5 to 10 mcg/kg per minute IV/IO.

Caution: Do not dilute in dextrose solution but can be co-infused with dextrose solutions.

Pediatric Advanced Life Support Drugs

Drug/Therapy	Indications/Precautions	Pediatric Dosage
Ipratropium Bromide	**Indications** Anticholinergic and bronchodilator used for treatment of asthma. **Precautions** • May cause pupil dilation if it enters eyes.	**Inhalation Dose** • 250 to 500 mcg (by nebulizer, MDI) every 20 minutes × 3 doses.
Lidocaine Can be given via endotracheal tube	**Indications** • Bolus therapy: — VF/pulseless VT. — Wide-complex tachycardia (with pulses). • RSI: May decrease ICP response during laryngoscopy. **Precautions/Contraindications** • High plasma concentration may cause myocardial and circulatory depression, possible CNS symptoms (eg, seizures). • Reduce infusion dose if severe CHF or low cardiac output is compromising hepatic and renal blood flow. • Contraindicated for bradycardia with wide-complex ventricular escape beats.	**VF/Pulseless VT, Wide-Complex Tachycardia (With Pulses)** **IV/IO:** • Initial: 1 mg/kg IV/IO loading dose. • Maintenance: 20 to 50 mcg/kg per minute IV/IO infusion (repeat bolus dose if infusion initiated >15 minutes after initial bolus therapy). **ET:** 2 to 3 mg/kg. **Rapid Sequence Intubation** 1 to 2 mg/kg IV/IO.

Magnesium Sulfate	Indications	Pulseless VT With Torsades
50% = 500 mg/mL	• Torsades de pointes or suspected hypomagnesemia.	25 to 50 mg/kg IV/IO bolus (maximum dose: 2 g).
	• Status asthmaticus not responsive to β-adrenergic drugs.	**Torsades (With Pulses), Hypomagnesemia**
	Precautions/Contraindications	25 to 50 mg/kg IV/IO (maximum dose: 2 g) over 10 to 20 minutes.
	• Contraindicated in renal failure.	**Status Asthmaticus**
	• Possible hypotension and bradycardia with rapid bolus.	25 to 50 mg/kg IV/IO (maximum dose: 2 g) over 15 to 30 minutes.
Milrinone	Indications	• Loading dose: 50 mcg/kg. Administer over 10 to 60 minutes. Monitor for hypotension.
	• Cardiogenic shock or heart failure marked by low contractility or high vascular resistance or both.	• Maintenance dose (continuous IV infusion): 0.25-0.75 mcg/kg per minute.
	Precautions/Contraindications	
	• May cause hypotension.	
	• May cause arrhythmias.	
	• Eliminated by renal excretion; use with caution in patients with renal insufficiency.	
	• Avoid in patients with ventricular outflow tract obstruction.	

Pediatric Advanced Life Support Drugs

Drug/Therapy	Indications/Precautions	Pediatric Dosage
Naloxone Can be given IV/IO/IM/subcutaneously Can be given via endotracheal tube; other routes preferred	**Indications** To reverse effects of narcotic toxicity: respiratory depression, hypotension, and hypoperfusion. **Precautions** • Half-life of naloxone often shorter than half-life of narcotic; repeated dosing is often required. • Administration to infants of addicted mothers may precipitate seizures or other withdrawal symptoms. • Assist ventilation before administration to avoid sympathetic stimulation. • May reverse effects of analgesics; consider administration of nonopioid analgesics for treatment of pain.	**Bolus IV/IO Dose** For *total* reversal of narcotic effects, give 0.1 mg/kg every 2 minutes PRN (maximum dose: 2 mg). *Note:* If total reversal is not required (eg, respiratory depression), smaller doses (0.001 to 0.005 mg/kg [1 to 5 mcg/kg]) may be used. Titrate to effect. **Continuous IV/IO Infusion** 0.002 to 0.16 mg/kg (2 to 160 mcg/kg) per hour IV/IO infusion.
Nitroglycerin	**Indications** • Heart failure (especially associated with myocardial ischemia). • Hypertensive emergency. • Pulmonary hypertension. **Precautions** • May cause hypotension, especially in hypovolemic patients.	**Dose (Continuous IV Infusion)** • Initial dose: 0.25-0.5 mcg/kg per minute. • Titrate by 1 mcg/kg per minute every 15-20 minutes. • Typical dose range: 1-5 mcg/kg per minute.

Nitroprusside
(Sodium Nitroprusside)

Mix in D_5W

Vasodilator that reduces tone in all vascular beds.

Indications

- Shock or low cardiac output states (cardiogenic shock) characterized by high vascular resistance.
- Severe hypertension.

Precautions

- May cause hypotension, particularly with hypovolemia.
- Metabolized by endothelial cells to cyanide, then metabolized in liver to thiocyanate and excreted by kidneys. Thiocyanate and cyanide toxicity may result if administered at high rates or with decreased hepatic or renal function. Monitor thiocyanate levels in patients receiving prolonged infusion, particularly if rate >2 mcg/kg per minute.
- Signs of thiocyanate toxicity include seizures, nausea, vomiting, metabolic acidosis, and abdominal cramps.

IV/IO Infusion

- 0.3 to 1 mcg/kg per minute initially; then titrate up to 8 mcg/kg per minute as needed.
- Light sensitive; cover drug reservoir with opaque material or use specialized administration set.
- Typically change solution every 24 hours.

Pediatric Advanced Life Support Drugs

Drug/Therapy	Indications/Precautions	Pediatric Dosage
Norepinephrine	Sympathetic neurotransmitter with inotropic effects. Activates myocardial β-adrenergic receptors and vascular α-adrenergic receptors. **Indications** [illegible] Treatment of shock and hypotension characterized by low systemic vascular resistance and unresponsive to fluid resuscitation. **Precautions** • May produce hypertension, organ ischemia, and arrhythmias. Extravasation may cause tissue necrosis (treat with phentolamine). • Do not administer in same IV tubing with alkaline solutions.	Begin at rates of 0.1 to 2 mcg/kg per minute; adjust infusion rate to achieve desired change in blood pressure and systemic perfusion.
Oxygen	**Indications** • Should be administered during stabilization of all seriously ill or injured patients with respiratory insufficiency, shock, or trauma even if oxyhemoglobin saturation is normal. • May monitor pulse oximetry to evaluate oxygenation and titrate therapy once child has adequate perfusion.	• Administer in highest possible concentration during initial evaluation and stabilization. • A nonrebreathing mask with reservoir delivers 95% oxygen with flow rate of 10 to 15 L/min. • After cardiac arrest, maintain oxyhemoglobin saturation 94%-99% (below 100%) to minimize risk of oxidative injury.

Procainamide	**Indications** SVT, atrial flutter, VT (with pulses). **Precautions** • Seek expert consultation when using this agent. • Routine use in combination with amiodarone (or other drugs that prolong QT interval) is not recommended without expert consultation. • Risk of hypotension and negative inotropic effects increases with rapid administration; not appropriate agent for VF/pulseless VT. • Reduce dose for patients with poor renal or cardiac function.	**Loading Dose** 15 mg/kg IV/IO over 30 to 60 minutes.
Prostaglandin E₁ **(PGE₁)** (Alprostadil)	**Indications** To maintain patency of ductus arteriosus in newborns with cyanotic congenital heart disease and ductal-dependent pulmonary or systemic blood flow. **Precautions** • May produce vasodilation, hypotension, apnea, hyperpyrexia, agitation, seizures. • May produce hypoglycemia, hypocalcemia.	**IV/IO Administration** • **Initial:** 0.05 to 0.1 mcg/kg per minute IV/IO infusion. • **Maintenance:** 0.01 to 0.05 mcg/kg per minute IV/IO infusion.

Pediatric Advanced Life Support Drugs

Drug/Therapy	Indications/Precautions	Pediatric Dosage

Sodium Bicarbonate
 	
8.4%: 1 mEq/mL in 10- or 50-mL syringe
 	
4.2%: 0.5 mEq/mL in 10-mL syringe
	Indications
	• Treatment of severe metabolic acidosis (documented or following prolonged arrest) unresponsive to ventilation and oxygenation.
	• Treatment of the following:
	  — Hyperkalemia.
	  — Sodium channel blocker toxicity, such as tricyclic antidepressants (after support of adequate airway and ventilation).
	
	Precautions
	• Routine administration is not recommended in cardiac arrest.
	• Infuse slowly.
	• Buffering action will produce carbon dioxide, so ventilation must be adequate.
	• Do not mix with any resuscitation drugs. Flush IV tubing with NS before and after drug administration.
	• Infiltration will cause tissue irritation.
		IV/IO Administration
		Metabolic Acidosis (Severe), Hyperkalemia
		IV/IO: 1 mEq/kg slow bolus.
		
		4.2% concentration recommended for use in infants <1 month of age.
		
		Sodium Channel Blocker Overdose (eg, Tricyclic Antidepressant)
		1 to 2 mEq/kg IV/IO bolus until serum pH is >7.45 (7.50 to 7.55 for severe poisoning) followed by IV/IO infusion of 150 mEq $NaHCO_3$/L solution to maintain alkalosis.

Vasopressin

Indications
- Cardiac arrest.
- Catecholamine-resistant hypotension.

Precautions
- Use with caution in patients with renal insufficiency or hyponatremia/free water overload.

- Cardiac arrest: 0.4-1 unit/kg IV/IO bolus (maximum dose: 40 units).
- Hypotension (continuous IV infusion): 0.0002-0.002 unit/kg per minute (0.2 to 2 milliunits/kg per minute).

Learn and Live® Through American Heart Association Programs

The American Heart Association has created a variety of programs and products for the public, healthcare professionals, and legislators that educate and raise awareness about cardiovascular health and disease prevention. Many also provide tools and information to help individuals and groups make an impact on improving survival in their communities. Learn more and get involved today.

Mission: Lifeline®

This national initiative seeks to improve the overall quality of care for ST-elevation myocardial infarction (STEMI) patients by improving systems of care. Learn more at www.Heart.org/MissionLifeline.

MISSION: LIFELINE®

Get With The Guidelines®

This suite of quality-improvement products empowers hospital teams to deliver heart and stroke care consistent with the most up-to-date scientific guidelines. To learn more, visit www.Heart.org/GetWithTheGuidelines.

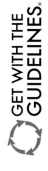

GET WITH THE GUIDELINES®

My Life Check™
Live Better With Life's Simple 7

My Life Check™/Life's Simple 7™
To help people improve their heart health, the AHA has developed an online resource, *My Life Check.* This short assessment easily identifies the AHA's defined "Simple 7" goals for ideal health and notes where a person is on the spectrum. Additional tools and information offer specific action steps to improve the measurements and track personal progress toward better health. Learn more at www.MyLifeCheck.Heart.org.

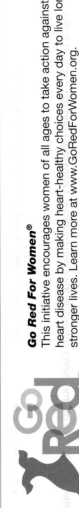

for women

Go Red TM of AHA, Red Dress TM of DHHS

Go Red For Women®
This initiative encourages women of all ages to take action against heart disease by making heart-healthy choices every day to live longer, stronger lives. Learn more at www.GoRedForWomen.org.

Learn about additional AHA programs at *www.Heart.org.*

Subject Labels

BLS	Rapid Sequence Intubation
Cardiac Arrest	Newborn Resuscitation
Bradycardia	Cyanotic Infant
Stable Tachycardia	PALS Rapid Sequence Intubation
Unstable Tachycardia	PALS Bradycardia
Stroke Algorithm	PALS Cardiac Arrest
Stroke Assessment	PALS Tachycardia— Poor Perfusion
Acute Coronary Syndromes	PALS Tachycardia— Adequate Perfusion
Fibrinolytic Checklist—STEMI	Trauma
12-Lead Changes	Routing Criteria for Injured Patient
Risk Stratification UA/NSTEMI	PALS Estimating ET Size/Depth
ACLS Drugs	PALS Drugs